# SpringerBriefs in Education

We are delighted to announce SpringerBriefs in Education, an innovative product type that combines elements of both journals and books. Briefs present concise summaries of cutting-edge research and practical applications in education. Featuring compact volumes of 50 to 125 pages, the SpringerBriefs in Education allow authors to present their ideas and readers to absorb them with a minimal time investment. Briefs are published as part of Springer's eBook Collection. In addition, Briefs are available for individual print and electronic purchase.

SpringerBriefs in Education cover a broad range of educational fields such as: Science Education, Higher Education, Educational Psychology, Assessment & Evaluation, Language Education, Mathematics Education, Educational Technology, Medical Education and Educational Policy.

SpringerBriefs typically offer an outlet for:

- An introduction to a (sub)field in education summarizing and giving an overview of theories, issues, core concepts and/or key literature in a particular field
- A timely report of state-of-the art analytical techniques and instruments in the field of educational research
- A presentation of core educational concepts
- An overview of a testing and evaluation method
- A snapshot of a hot or emerging topic or policy change
- An in-depth case study
- A literature review
- A report/review study of a survey
- An elaborated thesis

Both solicited and unsolicited manuscripts are considered for publication in the SpringerBriefs in Education series. Potential authors are warmly invited to complete and submit the Briefs Author Proposal form. All projects will be submitted to editorial review by editorial advisors.

SpringerBriefs are characterized by expedited production schedules with the aim for publication 8 to 12 weeks after acceptance and fast, global electronic dissemination through our online platform SpringerLink. The standard concise author contracts guarantee that:

- an individual ISBN is assigned to each manuscript
- each manuscript is copyrighted in the name of the author
- the author retains the right to post the pre-publication version on his/her website or that of his/her institution

Larrie Greenberg M.D.

# Misadventures in Patient Care and Medical Education

## Lessons Learned for the Clinician Educator

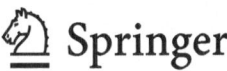 Springer

Larrie Greenberg M.D.
The George Washington University
School of Medicine and Health Sciences
Children's National Medical Center
Washington, DC, USA

ISSN 2211-1921          ISSN 2211-193X  (electronic)
SpringerBriefs in Education
ISBN 978-3-031-83929-0          ISBN 978-3-031-83930-6  (eBook)
https://doi.org/10.1007/978-3-031-83930-6

This Springer imprint is published by the registered company Springer Nature Switzerland AG
The registered company address is: Gewerbestrasse 11, 6330 Cham, Switzerland

If disposing of this product, please recycle the paper.

# Foreword

One is very fortunate in life when they meet an extraordinary person. I was so blessed when I met Larrie Greenberg. We were both the representatives from our schools to serve on the Association of American Medical Colleges (AAMC) steering committee for the Northeast Group on Educational Affairs. (NEGEA). We served side-by-side for years and bonded over our love for medical education and our fervent desire to improve as teachers and better help our learners learn.

Larrie was always a hero to me: a gifted teacher who loved the art and whose passion for teaching and the inspiration that emanated from him shone brightly. He had "the dream job" to my eye; he went to work with the sole purpose of enhancing education and through it, patient outcomes and provider satisfaction at his institution, the Children's National Medical Center and his school, George Washington University. Larrie had been walking the walk for years not only in his own institution but in the nation as he led the efforts to champion education in pediatrics and beyond. He was a role model for me and many others because he exuded his love for effective education, his profound substance in the science and practice of medical education and his ability to push the envelope, to apply educational principles in practice and to change the outcomes.

Larrie and I soon conspired to join together with his good friend, Rich Sarkin, a renowned pediatrician with a background prior to medicine as a middle school science teacher and later with Steve Miller, a pediatric ER doctor and another renowned educator to found a group we called the "Three Amigos" (even though there were four). This title was based on the silly movie of that name starring Steve Martin, Chevy Chase and Martin Short that came out at that time. Our group of Amigos conspired to do workshops at the AAMC meeting annually and later "on the road" by invitation. I was blessed to be a member with three pediatricians with both a love and flair for teaching. They exuded positivity, joy and inspiration. (I think it was in part because of the lessons from children they had learned in their own professional lives.) The Amigos developed almost a cult like following. It was so fun for us … and we were in the flow "zone" together enjoying our teaching and our connection to each other and the audience. We knew we were making a difference.

One of the last workshops we did together which served as the inspiration for this book was called "Not everything works in medical education." It was a huge success. I can still remember walking down the long corridor at the Washington Hilton where our workshop was to be held late on Tuesday afternoon, the last afternoon of the conference when many attendees had already gone home and others were "meeting-ed out." Our room was at the end of that corridor and the other rooms I passed with competing workshops had few attendees, but our room had people bursting out the doors with more in the corridors rushing to get in. The room was electric as we presented our own foibles, and I'll always remember when attendees began to read their own student critiques. After a particularly dreadful one, someone on the other side of the room would say "I can beat that" and read theirs. The feeling was cathartic but also as we unloaded our burdens, we began to support each other on how we could improve.

This experience was the impetus for this book. Teaching is a messy and difficult endeavor often fraught with blows to our self-esteem. Nobody does it perfectly all the time. We all can improve, and especially now as there are so many competing demands on both the teachers and learners. Parker Palmer has it pegged right....it takes courage to teach! (Parker J. Palmer, The Courage to Teach, Exploring the Inner Landscape of a Teacher's Life, Jossey-Boss, San Francisco, 1998).

Larrie shares many of his own painful lessons learned in this book, but in a way, his message is more about how to avoid these types of ego-deflating, sometimes humiliating, difficult to process experiences that all teachers go through.

My view is that the subtitle of this book might be "Larrie's wisdom, over a full life of impact on medical education." The word "wisdom" is important. The Greeks, especially Aristotle, had the notion that there were three buckets of things to learn. One was called "episteme" or knowledge, the reams of "stuff" that we had to learn. Another bucket was called "techne", or the skills we had to learn and a third was called "phronesis", often translated as "practical wisdom. The two former ones made up almost all the content of medical education. Phronesis was the hardest to teach. The authors Barry Schwartz and Ken Sharpe in their book Practical Wisdom said phronesis was doing the right thing in the right way at the right time for the right reason(s). (Barry Schwartz and Kenneth Sharpe, Practical Wisdom; the Right Way to do the Right Thing, Riverhead Books, 2011).

Wisdom has been called the "uber" virtue: a sort of orchestra leader, harmonizing all the other virtues. Dr. Margaret Plews-Ogan at the University of Virginia who runs the "Phronesis Project" there asks the question: "suppose wisdom was the guiding principle, the North Star, for our education? How different would education look then? Would it have a better chance in the formation of the "good physician?" My bet is so, and Larrie's pearls that follow can help us to see that "North Star" and practice phronesis.

One very interesting aspect of wisdom is that mistakes, misadventures and tough challenges are among the best proving grounds to develop wisdom. It has been said that: "good judgement comes from experience; and experience comes from bad judgement." At the most recent commencement ceremony at my institution (Dartmouth), the tennis great, Roger Federer, was the speaker. He asked the audience what percentage of points do you think he won in his career (with multiple Grand Slam wins)? The answer was a surprising 54%! He "failed" 46% of the time, yet still is one of the all time greats! Other famous speeches by J. K. Rowling at Harvard Commencement in 2008 and Steve Jobs highlighted the role of failure in their lives. When the former president of Dartmouth came from the school from the University of Michigan, he said if he had one wish for the students it would be "I wish they could learn to fail." His favorite course at Michigan was one on "clowning". At the beginning of the class, the students were asked to "be a clown" and get their classmates to laugh, but of course they failed. Then, the class taught them there were techniques and strategies, if you will, a "science" to clowning and at the end, they could be successful. The key to wisdom is how we learn from this adversity.

So, our workshop and subsequently this book come from lessons learned that we could be doing this better. The greatest enemy of wisdom is perfectionism!

In the last paragraph of the introduction, Larrie gives some suggestions on how to use the book. I would suggest heeding these, maybe even pasting them on a bulletin board or someplace easily and frequently seen. Try one new pearl a day. At the end of the year, you will have many new arrows in your quiver. Say to your learners: "This is a teaching point". "This is a feedback session—what do you think you did well? What can you improve? What opportunity do you have for improvement?" Say to yourself: "What do you see as an opportunity for educational scholarship? How do you find experts that can help with aspects or your paper in your institution?" Practice these skills: "Observe as you come into the room. Read the room. Recognize emotions"...... The list goes on and on.

One other message that I'd suggest you internalize is from the Rabbinical Jewish tradition is the wisdom from Pirkei Avot: "Get yourself a teacher, Acquire yourself a friend." Larrie is amazing teacher and now like he is to me, he is your friend. I am delighted to share him! His lessons are so heartfelt, genuine, practical and impactful. We all now have the gift of his compiled wisdom from a life well lived as a guy who went to work each day trying to improve education and was amazingly successful, especially at navigating bumps in the road and finding new cheese! (You'll get this reference as you read on!).

The Buddhists have an image of a little bird on your shoulder whispering in your ear words of advice. With the book and Larrie's pearls, we each have him on our shoulders whispering in our ears...... "think of doing this, rather than that" or "time to be silent" or......

As he ends the book with Robin Williams advice from the Dead Poets Society: Carpe diem. I'd like to encourage you all to Carpe EACH diem with Larrie! This will help each of us learn more and practice more phronesis.

Joseph F. O'Donnell, M.D.
Professor of Medicine and Psychiatry
(Emeritus)
The Geisel School of Medicine at
Dartmouth
Hanover, NH, USA

# Preface

This book is dedicated to my wonderful wife, Joyce, of 60 years who has shown the patience and support I have needed in my career as a Clinician Educator (CE). My work ethic was solid, and I always exclaimed that "I came to work the same time as the surgeons" and left late. This demanding schedule was my doing and based on my job description of founding and overseeing the Office at Medical Education at Children's National Medical Center in DC, one of the only offices in North America in the late 70s overseeing the full continuum of medical education, in addition to my clinical and other administrative responsibilities at Children's and the George Washington University School of Medicine and Health Sciences (GWU). Much of my creative thinking and educational scholarship (ES) was done in off-hours, namely at home at nights and weekends, as there was no protected time nor was I funded for these activities. Joyce always was there to support me, was the primary caregiver of our two successful and loving children (although I made it a point to be there for them for all special activities and during my time off) and was the social secretary, arranging meeting friends, attending the theater and leading the gardening effort in and outside our home. I owe so much to her as my career was long, busy and very fulfilling and importantly, I was able to include her at times in accompanying me to national and international meetings and being part of my professional life.

My parents were unbelievable in modeling and instilling in me caring, empathy, compassion, giving of themselves, looking after others and the meaning of family. They were always there for me and at an early age, allowed me to fly from the nest to explore and develop a sense of independence and responsibility.

I also dedicate this to my dear children, Abby, who inherited my Mother's artistic abilities and became a creative entrepreneur who makes beautifully decorated pretzels, candies and delicious truffles for parties, graduations and special occasions; and Jeff, a caring and committed pediatrician in practice who has been recognized for his teaching and patient care both in his practice and at Children's Hospital in DC; and their spouses: Shawn has a general law practice in the area and Stefanie is an elite gourmet cook who has previously worked in advertising and does a lot of volunteer work. I also am very proud of my grandchildren, whom I will list chronologically:

Josh, who graduated from the University of Virginia with a degree in architecture, received his master's degree in architecture from Parsons School of Design/The New School after being in the architectural workforce for three years; Bradley graduated from Virginia Tech in civil engineering and is working for Clark Construction, an international company; Jeremy graduated from the Kelly School of Business, Indiana University, and is working as a wealth management executive at Merrill Lynch; Adam graduated from Syracuse in the S. I. Newhouse School of Communications, but has changed his focus to outdoor and environmental interests; Jake is a third year at the University of Massachusetts; and Allie the same at University of Wisconsin. We have had a very special relationship with our grandchildren and consider ourselves fortunate to have been able to be part of their lives. Each is a special person in his/her own way, and we have been fortunate to have lived to this day to see their successes and struggles.

I also would like to thank leadership at Children's and GWU for having faith in me and allowing me to explore educational activities in the late 1970s when no one else was interested in education as a career focus. I was able to attend educational meetings at the Association of American Medical Colleges (AAMC) in addition to the American Educational Research Association (AERA), the latter of which consists of research from elementary school all the way up to the professions. In those early years, professional societies like pediatrics, internal medicine and other major specialty groups did not focus on education as a major component of national meetings or journals, and early CEs presented and published their work in educationally oriented journals versus their specialty journals. Thus, it was appropriate and logical that my initial mentors were Ph.Ds. who populated medical schools in deans' offices and research divisions and were active nationally as there were no educational role models in my department or medical school. To emphasize my point about the dearth of CEs who focused on education in those early days, I recall presenting a poster on the effects of a continuing professional education series on the performance of practicing physicians at a Pediatric national meeting and was the **only** educational offering in the entire poster session. That has so changed with time!

Lastly, I am indebted to all those educators along the way that enabled my career, mentoring me, sharing their successes and failures and just being there as wonderful colleagues. In my recently published *Primer* for the CE, I sought no outside expertise in writing that book. In this current endeavor, however, recognizing this was uncharted territory in terms of gleaning limited information from previously published books and articles about the topics, I recognized the need to reach out and solicit expertise from colleagues on these areas. In that vein, I want to recognize 6 valued colleagues and friends who provided input on different sections of the book: Janet Fischel, Ph.D., Emeritus Professor Pediatrics, Renaissance University at Stony Brook School of Medicine, who provided some insights on educational scholarship: Karen Wendelberger Marcdante, M.D., Professor Emeritus (deceased), Medical College of Wisconsin, who commented on a number of areas; Janet Serwint, M.D., Professor Emeritus of Pediatrics Johns Hopkins University School of Medicine, who provided terrific thoughts about mentoring; W. Scott Schroth, MD, MPH, former Associate Dean for Administration, GWU who advised me on administrative issues; Ben Siegel, M.D., Professor of Pediatrics and Psychiatry, Boston University School of Medicine, retired Pediatrician, Boston Medical Center contributed to the patient care section; and Arnie Schwartz, M.D., Ph.D. former Associate Dean of Faculty Affairs and Professor Emeritus of Pathology, who contributed to the tenure and promotion section.

These are and have been dear colleagues, most of whom I have met as fellow clerkship directors in pediatrics when I was one of the founders of the Council on Medical Student Education in Pediatrics (COMSEP); others through my pediatric academic home, the Academic Pediatric Association; some through Children's and/or through my activities at GWU. These are fellow CEs with whom I have dined, commiserated, collaborated and shared stories of personal and professional interest. In essence, life-long colleagues that I have valued over the years for their friendship and expertise in medical education, administration and patient care. All I can say is "Thank you for being there."

I have been fortunate to have published over 7 decades, my first paper being in the late 60s and now in the 2020s I have published a number of articles, the *Primer* and now this book. I consider myself fortunate, in my career, to have been a small part of the medical educational community who was responsible for helping to be a formative force through interactions, mentorship, collaborations, coaching and counseling the current generation of educators.

Potomac, USA                                                              Larrie Greenberg M.D.

# Contents

# Chapter 1
# Introduction

In 2022 I published a *Primer* focused on the clinician educator, those academic faculty in medicine and health sciences that assume the major responsibility for teaching, patient care, educational scholarship, advocacy and mentoring in our academic health centers. That publication triggered an idea for this book; i.e., reflecting on mistakes clinician educators make in patient care and with their educational responsibilities. Historically, there have been just a few publications that have addressed mistakes specifically made by physicians in patient care, the most important of which was the 1999 Institute of Medicine's treatise *To Err is Human: Building a Safer Health System,* which recognized how errors impact the safety of patients. This report stated there were 44,000–98,000 preventable deaths each year due to errors in the health-care system, a number that is quite overwhelming considering the perspective that the Ohio State football stadium holds about 103,000 people. This concern about patient safety led to President Clinton signing the Senate bill that authorized the Health-care Research and Quality Act of 1999 to address these preventable errors. Another impactful publication was Jerome Groopman's book on *How Doctors Think,* which presented information to decipher how physicians problem-solve in different areas of medicine as they decide what the patient's problem(s) are and how to address those. He provides interesting examples how physicians in different specialties can make mistakes when dealing with patients. These publications are very patient-oriented and some of the root causes of mistakes in medicine seem to gravitate to miscommunication or lack of communication with patients. Interesting that it has taken medicine a long time to address errors in patient care through quality improvement (QI) projects, morbidity and mortality rounds and through legal offices imbedded in our institutions.

On the education side of this equation, I fondly recall presenting a peer-reviewed workshop at the Association of American Medical Colleges in 1994 with Dr. Joseph O'Donnell, a superb educator and oncologist from Dartmouth Medical School and Dr. Rich Sarkin, a consummate generalist and educationalist in Pediatrics from The Jacobs School of Medicine and Biomedical Sciences at the University of Buffalo

© The Author(s), under exclusive license to Springer Nature Switzerland AG 2025
L. Greenberg M. D., *Misadventures in Patient Care and Medical Education*,
SpringerBriefs in Education, https://doi.org/10.1007/978-3-031-83930-6_1

on misadventures in medical education, the title of which I have incorporated in this book. We had never seen anything preceding our workshop that addressed the 'mea culpa' approach in education nor did we know what the reception of educators would be to this topic. Not exaggerating, there were not enough chairs in the room to accommodate all participants that wanted to be in this workshop and the doors to the room were kept open so those who couldn't get seating could see/hear the discussion from the hallway. Based on this experience, I surmised there was a keen interest in this topic and fellow educators wanted to hear about the faux pas to which the three of us confessed. Hence, this area will be the major focal and discussion point in the book.

Like the aforementioned *Primer*, this book will not be laden with an exhaustive list of references but rather selected references that add value to the discussion. I have divided the book into the following chapters, with the focus on mistakes we make in each of these areas: Patient Care, Educational Scholarship, Teaching, Administration, Promotion and Tenure and Mentorship. I also address how one can recognize these errors and suggest paths to correct them. In essence, mistakes can be important as a part of the scientific process, especially as we learn from them. Unlike the *Primer*, narrative stories will be a very small part of this book and bulleted topics will be the layout. Whereas I list what I would consider common mistakes in each category, these are not all-encompassing, and I am certain readers can add to these lists and enhance the discussion by identifying additional mistakes and reflecting on what we can do better. In addition, it is not predictable who the readership will be and how pertinent these lists will be for any specific reader. Finally, I have not provided an in-depth introductory treatise on each of the six areas I am addressing in that there are other publications; namely books, book chapters and scientific and peer-reviewed descriptive articles that do that quite well in defining these topics in much more significant detail. I refer the reader to those publications for more description on these topics. In addition, faculty who address some of the major topics with colleagues and/or trainees can engender areas which I omitted for further discussion.

I also realize that there is some overlap between this book and the *Primer* I have published in 2022, but the large majority of areas I discuss are new to this publication. I have re-emphasized some points I made in the Primer and re-look at them without accompanying stories. I also know that when there is no preceding literature on which to build when writing a book, there will be some gaps and omissions that are not always so obvious to the author. In essence, I hope clinician educators in medicine and health sciences enjoy the read and more importantly, learn from many of the examples and apply them to their practices. One important caveat in this publication not mentioned in my previous book is that senior students in medicine and health sciences would benefit from reading aspects of this book as they prepare for residency training and practice. Looking at errors in patient care, teaching and other areas might help students avoid these misadventures knowing them ahead of time. And, I hope with this publication I have brought awareness to the topic and have encouraged discussions in your own institutions, on points I have and have not decided to narrate. All institutions have morbidity and mortality conferences that address mistakes in addition to examining the results of QI studies that identify gaps and strengths in our performance. These are but two examples of how we have learned to identify and address mistakes, especially in patient care. It is less likely that misadventures in medical education have been found elsewhere in detail and listing these was fun, based on experiences and observations in the clinical setting, and noting some literature in specific areas. Lastly, we are all likely to have made make mistakes over the years we spend in training and in practice and it is hopeful, through prospective and retrospective reflection, we are able to 'correct' those errors so that our learners and patients are not harmed, and that exercise in reflective thinking becomes part of our growth as healthcare providers in academic medicine. These critical incidents also allow us to reflect on issues that 'went wrong' versus celebrating those that were successes......and learn from them.

My suggestions going through the book are: (1) Danger...this is not for bedtime reading; (2) Share thoughts and reflections with colleagues to hear each other's takes on topics and learn from them; (3) Think about what the practical applicability the major teaching points are in the clinical setting, and strategies to inculcate them covertly into the curriculum; (4) Look for bumps in the road that are likely going to be challenging in going from Point A to Point B and how one might traverse or by-pass those bumps; (5) Think about it is as a process to stir emotions and discussion; allow creativity to reach its closure, however that is defined; and collaborate as to how to approach a problem; and (6) Read contextually. If you are focusing on improving your teaching, read that section first. Discussion in groups creates new ideas and approaches that seem viable processes to effectively address the problem. In other words, I am asking that you try techniques to discuss the book in more detail, bringing ideas perhaps not specifically listed in the book. Rich discussions should evolve on topics in and not in the book that can make for a wonderful learning experiences based on timely topics noted. This approach is in-synch with the principles John Dewey, one of the fathers of contemporary education, espoused over a century ago; i.e., the learner needs to be proactive in learning.

# Chapter 2
# Teaching

Teaching is one of the most important responsibilities of the academic clinician educator and the one that attracts many faculty into the academic setting. None of us in the field are 'born teachers,' although there are personality traits that enable teachers to connect to learners in a more effective manner. It need not have to be said that there is a body of knowledge around teaching and learning that we as CEs all need to master. As we enter academic medicine or health sciences, availing ourselves to workshops that address teaching and learning in addition to self-directed learning on these topics enables us to understand the principles of teaching and learning and apply those in the clinical setting. There is also an important division between the scholarship of teaching and teaching excellence, which I will address in the section on ES. I use teaching in the context of the different venues to convey information to trainees and colleagues, in addition to interactive activities that promote learning. I am including a list of possible mistakes in teaching with suggestions on how to recognize and overcome these. As I reflected on the volume of information I have written on each section of this book, it seems that teaching received slightly more of my attention than other areas. Whereas I was totally invested in patient care and saw myself as a committed and thorough caregiver (often being asked by colleagues to see their patients around a specific problem), I became absorbed in the process of teaching and learning early on, reading voraciously about the underpinnings of these issues as they apply to the clinical setting. Much of my initial reading was not from the medical field but from the education field from which undergraduate students learn to be teachers!!! In Pediatrics I was one of the first CEs to devote my career devoted to the process of how learners learn and how faculty should teach.

There is a wonderful saying in Pirkei Avot 1:6, Chapters or Ethics of our Fathers, a compilation of the ethical teachings and maxims from Rabbinic Jewish tradition, that says 'Get yourself a teacher, acquire for yourself a friend.' Whereas teachers and learners do not necessarily become friends, they can have a bond and connectedness that results from a safe learning climate. When a teacher observes an enthusiastic learner, it reinforces the process and makes it so much more worthwhile. Summarily,

L. Greenberg M. D., *Misadventures in Patient Care and Medical Education*, SpringerBriefs in Education, https://doi.org/10.1007/978-3-031-83930-6_2

when the learner resonates with a teacher, this often promotes learning to a high level often not predictable. In essence, it becomes a mutual admiration society. Now, on to the misadventures in teaching. These are not listed in a specific order and I tried to organize them so that related topics followed one another.

- Designating feedback as positive or negative is a misnomer. Everyone needs feedback in their workplace and the feedback we give/receive should be regarded as reinforcing for things we do well and corrective for those that need fine-tuning (Hewson & Little, 1998). That should be made clear to learners at the beginning of any rotation via an orientation; i.e., that feedback will be given on a regular basis in the format of both corrective and reinforcing and should be received in that mindset. It seems our culture has sensitized people in general to be told 'You did a great job', with very little to inform that person what did they do that was so great and just as importantly, what could they improve. That said, I often heard students and trainees complaining that they always seemed to be evaluated. We should emphasize early in a rotation that we give feedback because we care about our trainees and want them to grow and be the best they can be on our watch and beyond. Many faculty still look at feedback in the traditional way of positive and negative, with the latter connotation having a possible harmful impact on the learner. Once faculty tell the learner what they have done well, the learner then awaits the 'bad news' using this model. In fact, corrective feedback should not be looked upon as negative but what we should all seek to become better physicians and healthcare providers through the feedback process. Learners in a trusting environment look for feedback on what they have done well and what can be improved although the feedback process should never be assumed but addressed as an integral part of the rotation in an orientation. Trainees should feel empowered in a safe learning climate to request feedback from faculty and/or residents following patient interactions, being proactive in patient care, leading a team in discussion of a patient, etc.
- Feedback can focus on what the trainee needs to improve and need not address what she has done well. It is important for trainees to hear about what they have performed well so they are aware of continuing that behavior in the future. As a clerkship director for 22 years, I often saw faculty writing summative evaluations that included behaviors that the trainee needed to improve, omitting those the trainee did well. I sent those narratives back to faculty to suggest they add the information about what they observed the trainee doing well. Balancing corrective and reinforcing feedback is ideal as there are always teaching points to relay to the trainee in either of these areas. Paying attention to what the learner does well (as part of the competencies/milestones) is important to record in addition to mentioning what needs improvement. This balance of summative feedback is important for the trainee to hear, read and digest. What is written should be a carbon copy of what faculty relate to the trainee in-person; i.e., verbal feedback, which sometimes doesn't happen according to trainees' experiences.
- Giving effective feedback takes too much time. In my experience locally and nationally, this has often been a concern of faculty over the years in that they are

busy and don't feel they can squeeze feedback into the interaction with the trainee. In fact, we can teach effective feedback skills and demonstrate that this important function takes very little time. The SOAP model developed by my colleague at GWU, Jim Blatt, M.D. starts with 'How do you think things went?' The usual reply is 'I think I did fine' (Chokshi et al., 2023). The follow-up is 'Tell me what you think you did well and what you can improve upon.' After that interaction, the teacher then states, 'This is what I saw you doing well and this is what you can fine-tune.' Then, the teacher-learner explore ways to go forward in the future to make subsequent interactions with patients even better; i.e., having the trainee generate learning objectives for future similar interactions. In my experience observing residents over a number of years, the feedback process consumed a very small part of the interaction, usually less than 3–5 min (Greenberg, 2020, pp. 569–574). Teaching this skill has been the focus of many innovative workshops and scholarly papers over the last 25 years.

- Not making feedback part of a humanistic habit. Being consistent with feedback is critical to a trainee's growth and as mentioned, the time it takes even in a very busy clinical environment is not significant over the course of a day. These skills of giving feedback, no matter what model is employed, are an important part of faculty growth and assuring that trainees receive the feedback they deserve. The shortest word in the English language that contains the letters a, b, c, d, e and f happens to be feedback. Without, it makes the road to success that much harder for any of us.

- Not searching the literature for ways to enhance the feedback you give. As faculty, many of us have been exposed to ways to give effective feedback through workshops, modeling and personal experience. There are evidence-based ways to provide effective feedback that can go unnoticed. One describes a clinical encounter card (CEC) that we used in our ambulatory area as a way to enhance and increase feedback to medical students (Greenberg, 2004). We conducted a workshop to orient faculty to this methodology, with the agreement that after each interaction with a student, faculty would record on the CEC their assessment of how the student performed. Using the card, they would then engage the student and relate their assessment of the student with that patient. In turn, if faculty did not engage the student, the student was also provided a CEC and approached the faculty member to provide feedback. Students reported that feedback increased significantly in the ambulatory rotation, more so than other clinical rotation. Using evaluation methods with Likert scales alone to measure the effectiveness of our teaching is not the most effective way to assess how we teach. When trainees evaluate our teaching, they need to write in a narrative fashion in addition to circling numbers from 1 to 5 on reflections about our teaching. It is so typical of trainees to circle all 5s (representing 'excellent') on an evaluation form provided by the department or medical school and not include any comments about our performance as to why we deserved all 5s. This kind of feedback is not particularly helpful to faculty who often are seeking ways to improve how they teach their learners. Narratives, on the other hand, can provide more useful information that reinforces and/or helps the teacher in future encounters. I have advocated for the Brookfield Critical Incident Questionnaire, which Brookfield has employed in classroom teaching but can be used in the clinical setting. Brookfield poses 5 questions: When were you most engaged in the teaching interaction? When were you most distanced? What action did your peers or the teacher take that was most affirmative or helpful? What action was most confusing or puzzling? And what was most surprising? (Brookfield, 1995). Using this evaluation model or variation thereof can provide the teacher with more specifics and detailed information about his teaching. The questionnaire can promote trust, empowerment, growth and diversity of learners. I amended the Brookfield model while observing residents and medical students as a volunteer over an 18-year period at Children's Hospital (Greenberg, 2020, pp. 1–6, Aug 2020). Every resident I observed completed this two-questionnaire form, completing it anonymously. Their responses provided me with insights into what they had learned and how they perceived their interaction with me.

- Not making a clear division between patient care issues versus teaching. Over time in my career, I have found that trainees have sometimes stated that 'There was no teaching on rounds or in the ambulatory setting'. In fact, almost all of our teaching is conducted within the context of patient care and that is what makes it so poignant and pertinent, an adult learning principle at its best. Trainees confuse the narrative on what is patient-care related and what is teaching and in fact, they can be one-in-the-same. I am suggesting as what we published in the 8-step preceptor (Ottolini et al., 2010) that you announce your teaching point(s) perhaps using the following language, 'I want to make a teaching point', alerting trainees to that happening. That helps divide what the learner might determine is patient care 'talk' versus teaching. This attention to teaching in the midst of intensive patient care activities can guide the learner as to how teaching is occurring within the context of patient care and alerting the learner that a teaching point is coming. This model may seem awkward at first but making it part of your being while teaching can be helpful in how learners differentiate patient care versus teaching points.

- Not being perceptive about trainee learning styles/preferences. Whereas learners have preferences in the way they learn depending on the situation, teachers need to recognize that when there are pauses after the teacher asks questions, those pauses reflect many underlying issues: like (1) no previous experience with a similar patient, (2) no previous knowledge on that topic, (3) disorganization in thinking, (4) hesitancy to commit oneself, or (5) synthesizing one's approach in concert with her preferred learning styles. An example of the latter is the following scenario: 'Can you tell me the anatomic structure of the Circle of Willis?' Illustrating my point, the student response could be, 'I can't verbalize that but I can draw it for you.' There are many learning styles/preferences inventories and I have used Rezler's Learning Preference Inventory since she mentored me briefly when I was visiting the Center for Educational Development at the University of Illinois in the 70s (Jewett et al., 1985). Whereas we cannot always recognize every learner's learning styles for each patient, reframing questions when the learner is not able to answer can sometimes alert us to how each learner addresses a particular situation.

Reflecting on my own learning styles, I score high in the abstract category on Rezler's Learning Preference Inventory BUT in some situations, I rely on concrete thinking or a group approach versus working independently to solve a problem. So, our learning preferences vary as to the context in which they occur and the teacher needs to be aware of those when questioning the learner. Just asking learners how they seem to learn best is a great start!

- There is no time to teach. I often hear this comment made by hospitalists and ambulatory care physicians working in extremely busy settings, similar to their responses on feedback. This likely also occurs with health science faculty. I understand this response but in fact, teaching can take a matter of seconds, meaning that one can make poignant teaching points even 'on-the-run' in a brief period of time. I always wonder when faculty make this comment about teaching, perhaps they are referring to a traditional hour-long more formal and scheduled teaching session. Basically, it is not about the amount of time one teaches. It's about being consistent and making at least one teaching point on each patient. Trainees seem to appreciate consistency of teaching and almost never comment about the amount of time we teach. The take-home point is thinking consciously about teaching on each patient, even if it happens walking down a corridor to see the next patient in the hospital or exiting a room where you and the trainee have interacted around a patient. Again, the 8-step preceptor, initially aimed at ambulatory teaching, emphasizes efficiency and can be a 5-min interaction with the trainee. I maintain more is not better! Engage the learner, find out what his/her experience is with similar patients, and make teaching points based on that information which can be obtained very quickly. I have made this point in the *Primer; i.e.,* everyone on the team is a teacher. Make certain you delegate teaching responsibilities to give everyone on the team an opportunity to share their knowledge and teaching style. I remember to this day when an ambulatory fellow (General Pediatrics), responsible for leading a teaching session as part of the rotation in medical education, taught about the differences between Old and New World wines, bringing in examples of those wines and cheeses to help reinforce the tastes of both. It was an 'aha' moment for me. I wouldn't have gotten the differences had she not actually had us taste the wines accompanied by cheeses. This was creative and innovative teaching, translating the abstract into actual examples by tasting. And the time for learners to recognize the differences was short and to the point.

- Teachers may not know the level of the learners whom they will be engaging. The teacher may assume what needs to be taught or might decide to discuss her favorite research topic for an assigned teaching session. In general, that is such a mistake and can leave learners not engaged and distanced. Connecting the dots on knowing who your learners are can be tricky, especially when it comes to lecturing to a larger group. Whoever invites you to speak needs to let you know what he/she thinks the level of the audience is on a particular topic especially an educational one. Often, I hear back that most of the audience will have had little to no experience with adult learning and education and that my comments should be directed to the lowest common denominator knowledge-wise. As a specific example of determining the level of your learners, I had an experience at a national meeting where my good friend and colleague Rich Sarkin and I were facilitating a workshop, planned in advance by email. As we started the workshop and had participants vocalize what their experiences were with our topic, Rich and I independently were amazed at the advanced level of the audience and took a brief time-out to redesign and transform the workshop spontaneously into a train-the-trainer session, where participants could facilitate the workshop in their home institutions. This flexibility is critical to assure the session will be meaningful to the learners, once one has established where the learners are around a specific topic. Again, knowing your learners when you are engaging a large group is important and when you are dealing with individual learners, asking them if they have ever previously seen a patient like this is a way to determine the level of the learner. On occasion the more senior residents, when asked, will respond they have seen many patients like this previously. When I hear that, I then usually ask how I can be helpful on this particular patient. In fact, that question raises antennae in residents as they are seldom IF EVER asked that question and usually hesitate to answer. If that is the case, be prepared to follow-up with a suggestion or two.

- The absence of an orientation that includes information in writing on a website **and** verbally, highlighting important issues for that rotation is a mistake, violating adult learning principles. A well-thought-out orientation for trainees on a specific rotation and/or clerkship can lay out where the journey is heading for the next number of weeks. As the infamous New York Yankee Hall of Fame catcher Yogi Berra once said, 'If you don't know where you are going, you will wind up some-place else.' In this regard, I have often been confronted with a statement like 'the residents don't seem interested in this rotation.' My first reaction is 'What do you tell them in an orientation?' It is frequently mentioned that there is no orientation. Therefore, when trainees are not certain about ground rules, learning experiences, roles, responsibilities, expectations and the feedback/evaluation process, they can tend to show disinterest or even confusion. This lack of clear goals, responsibilities, roles and expectations can result in trainees having angry feelings, dismissing this rotation as not important (and the content might well be important in their future practice), and giving mixed 'signals' to faculty. Malcolm Knowles, in his classic work on adult learning examining non-healthcare people in the workforce, suggested a learning contract to activate learners and have them express their own learning needs for a particular experience. For example, the trainee can state that for this rotation, 'I want to learn specifically how to examine the tympanic membrane and decipher acute ear infections from chronic ear problems'. This process can inform faculty what the learning needs are of the trainee and navigate how the trainee can accomplish those goals. Half-way through the rotation, it is appropriate to revisit these goals and determine how well the trainee is accomplishing them, with faculty facilitating the session. I would end this section on a positive note to say that there are many trainees who have been long-time achievers and they will master the content and skills of a given rotation with or without us!! So, learning can go on without the teacher (not ideal, unless the teacher is present as a non-entity) but cannot go on without the learner!

- Not translating creative knowledge and skills into workshops. This has been a focus for and a passion for me over time. I have enjoyed collaborating with colleagues creating educational workshops that teach colleagues specific knowledge and skills that they can use immediately in the workplace. Submitting these workshops for acceptance at national meetings is another form of educational activities to be included in an educator portfolio. I get a feeling of fulfillment when I know I have contributed to colleagues' expertise by introducing them to concepts like adult learning theory, communication issues, and teaching innovations. For me, the value of these collaborations has been meeting new and creative faculty from all over North America who have brought such wonderful approaches to different topics in education. I acknowledge Sarah Forgie, M.D., current Dean of the College of Medicine, the University of Saskatchewan, who has been so creative in teaching infectious diseases to medical students, residents and peers through music from Dave Brubeck's *Take Five* song, magic from Harry Houdini, and puppets. I had the privilege of facilitating a couple of workshops with her at our national pediatric meetings and the learning that occurred in those workshops through laughter and collegiality among participants who had not met previously was so contagious that the noise level impacted participants in other workshops in the vicinity. Fellow pediatricians were asking what was going on 'in the room where it happened', to borrow a song title from *Hamilton*. Colleagues approached me with smiles stating they heard the cacophony. Who said learning can't be fun!! Sarah's creativity captures how learning can be constructed to be enjoyable and memorable by learners.

  Some of my teaching that has evolved into interactive and challenging workshops that have been presented in visiting professorships and peer-reviewed national meetings include the 8-step preceptor (cased-based teaching), the problem learner, brief, structured observation, adult learning principles and questioning skills.

- Not appropriately and objectively documenting a potential professional issue about a learner is an error. Sometimes we see aberrant behavior or performance by a trainee that has not been noted before (documented in discussions with the residency training program or clerkship directors). There is a tendency, in my experience, locally and nationally, to view this behavior or performance as likely isolated and perhaps not needing reporting. I would suggest this is a grievous error and one that might come back to haunt the medical center if one of our graduates harms patients or participates in devious behavior contrary to the standards of practice. Whereas this problem could be isolated and may never occur again, indeed this could be the first occurrence **that faculty have noticed** this problem and it could be an ongoing issue not previously recognized. When I counsel a trainee and state my concerns about her performance, I listen to the trainee before making any judgment calls. I always state that this behavior or performance is not acceptable; i.e., below expectations, and that I will state so in my summative evaluation. I also point out that if this is something that has occurred in the past and not recognized or reported previously by faculty, it is a serious issue that the trainee needs to address. I have seen issues like not keeping to timelines or communicating as requested on educational scholarship projects, abusive behavior of nurses that uncovered a trainee's substance abuse, learning disabilities not previously recognized manifested in organizational skills dysfunction and faulty problem-solving, tardiness in appearing in designated clinical assignments, and lying to cover up performance issues that were a result of alcohol abuse as a few examples. In our institution (GWU), past deans responsible for medical students on clinical rotations have omitted aberrant behavior from letters for residency application **if** indeed these incidents were isolated. With residents and health science students, faculty have an opportunity to observe them over 3–7 years and have an opportunity to determine if unacceptable behaviors or performance are repetitive. Bottom line: If you see something concerning about a trainee's performance, report that issue after discussing it with the trainee. Once the problem is agreed upon by both the CE and the trainee, then it is up to the latter to determine how he is going to improve that behavior and over what period of time. Some issues might require immediate and temporary dismissal from the program while the trainee receives the appropriate therapy, such as substance abuse.

- Looking at a group and assuming who is the teacher and who are the learners. When medical schools evolved in North America based on the British/European system of medical education, the model we adapted to American medicine originally was very hierarchical. As in the British system, professors were revered and their teaching was not generally interactive but more top-down. Professors, so easily identified in a group or dyad settings, seemed often unapproachable and far removed from trainees in their interactions and teaching. Many of us have traversed the current hierarchy in medicine as we have gone from trainee to faculty. It's almost as if we are members of a fraternity/sorority and that those at the top get to harass those at the bottom, since the same kinds of harassment and events happened to them!! We sometimes think of CEs as **the** teachers in a group as opposed to everyone having something educationally to offer. In parallel models outside of medicine, apprenticeship programs seem to be more user-friendly to the trainee, a system where the 'student' works by the side of the electrician or carpenter and eventually gets to demonstrate his competence and creativity through his work. That work continues until the apprentice has reached a specific level of competency that was determined at the beginning of the relationship. There are some physical determinants in healthcare, the short white coats for students, the long white coats for faculty (if they wear white coats!!) and residents can be anywhere in between that seem to delineate who is who on the team. Well, adult learning theory has transformed that notion and I would suggest the following: (1) We are all learners and that concept is an integral part of our commitment to continuing professional education. There is not a time when faculty are not learning in parallel with trainees about patient problems and new ways to teach. (2) The teachers in the group are not just those that look older and might be wearing that long coat. It is sometimes much better for faculty to be a scribe on the side than a sage on the stage; i.e., the faculty enable teaching to happen from those on the team! Trainees bring so much experience from their past, some as healthcare workers, others as patients or involved with patients and/or family members as patients; and as faculty, if we only gave them a chance to lead and share these experiences, we would all benefit. This is also a way to activate learners and give them permission to be a vibrant part of the team. That permission has to be emphasized in orientation and periodically again if we see trainees holding back. (3) Lastly, I explain to trainees the major professional difference between me and them is basically my long years of experience. Through those experiences, I have obtained new knowledge and skills which I continue to apply to my patients and teaching. In other words, there is a gap between learners and me age- and experience-wise; but that is not the typical hierarchical gap that the English and European system afforded the professor as compared to HIS (there were no HERS) lowly colleagues. This relationship of faculty to trainees I tried to convey here is part of a safe learning climate in which trainees thrive because they emotionally sense the collaborative effect and effort of faculty using this model. So, be collaborative with trainees.

- Not setting a safe learning climate. This was one of Knowles's adult learning principles in the workplace and it eventually filtered down to classroom teaching, looking at the environment (heated or air conditioned appropriately, seating conducive to interactive discussion [e.g., if you are conducting a workshop, arriving an hour ahead of time and arranging the seating based on how you will be conducting the workshop is paramount], room ideally with light coming from the outside), and the teacher's inter-connectedness to the learners. In the clinical setting, additional principles for setting a safe learning climate is to make certain the goals and objectives are clear for the teaching session or rotation, that you learn the names of participants as best you can, use 'I' comments that convey that you have been down this same path the learners are going ('I can remember when I was a trainee and having to perform a procedure I had never done before.'), point out likely learning experiences on the rotation, define the role of the learner, setting a tone that suggests a safe learning environment, establishing a 'positive' first impression, and being collegial as mentioned above. The learning climate perceptions begin with the initial interaction between teachers and learners so making it 'right' from the start is critical. In academic medicine, we tend to do things over and over, like orientations, and we need to be cognizant that whereas this repetition might be at times boring for us, this is a new experience for the learners, as they are entering the system for the first time. In summary, we should approach each initial interaction with learners with enthusiasm, treat this as if this was the first time presenting the information, and convey our commitment to the field. This sets the tone for the rest of the rotation with them.
- The teacher is doing most of the talking. Jerry Harvey, a well-known organizational management guru from George Washington University (Harvey, 1979) expressed some wonderful thoughts about teaching and learning. He implied that when he was talking, he was never certain his students were learning! Conversely, when there was cacophony in a lecture room, he was certain learning was occurring as the students were doing the talking. In any interaction with learners other than lecturing (I will address that later), I am always conscious of teacher talk versus learner talk. If the latter is doing most of the talking, it is easier for the teacher to assess the learner's knowledge and problem-solving skills as opposed to the

well-meaning teacher monopolizing the interaction, as is sometimes the case. When we 'talk at someone', we can never be certain whether or not that person is learning and more importantly, don't know what he is learning! So, when you are teaching, think about the teacher-talk time versus how much the learners are talking. If you are doing most of the talking, it's likely there is not a lot of learning going on. Parenthetically, I realize that the zealous and committed teacher wants to share of her knowledge and experience with learners, but just remember these interactions are not about the teacher!!!

- Taking responsibility for what others learn. That is never the job of the teacher! The teacher is there to facilitate learning and make connections based on experiences the learner may not have. It might be antithetical to what our educational system is about, but in fact, learners do not always need teachers to learn but teachers always need learners to teach. That said, I see our role to be value-added to what the learner is already absorbing from their reading and patient experiences. We should be the facilitators to help bring some of these issues; i.e., book learning and clinical experiences, together. The challenge for all learners is to set personal clear goals on what and how they learn during a specific rotation, of course in context with the overall goals and objectives prescribed for the rotation. As teachers, we should be aware of their goals and help learners to have opportunities to achieve them. Hopefully, expectations are made clear early on, with learners accepting those challenges and many going beyond what is expected. Reading on each patient for whom they care is something I always required so that the learner could demonstrate to me that he was learning within the context of patient care. The learner who is not meeting expectations is one that likely has a problem that needs addressing, whether that be affective, cognitive interpersonal or structural in origin.

- Not including reflection as part of your teaching. Ever since Dewey introduced the concept of reflection in 1933, Donald Schon continued his work and has written extensively about reflection. In my opinion, it should be a humanistic habit that we all incorporate into our teaching and patient care. Schon envisioned reflection as in-action and on-action, while others extended that theory into reflection-for-action (Farrell, 2013). Reflection represents a powerful tool as part of our teaching (Plack & Greenberg, 2005). So, applying this concept to teaching starts as a conscious exercise as one engages trainees and/or peers. Eventually this becomes an unconscious effort that becomes part of your being. Reflection can occur in so many different teaching venues. In a large lecture hall, I never stand behind the podium but request a roving microphone so that I can teach by walking, up and down the aisles, and observing faces as I speak. I am also conscious in these large group sessions of time and often eliminate the end of my planned session to accommodate questions and comments from the audience. In one-on-one teaching interactions or smaller groups, it is easier to assess if learners are engaged and on some occasions, I will ask 'You don't seem to be engaged' or 'I don't seem to be connecting to you.' This happens prospectively and is labeled reflection-in-action. The notion of reflection-on-action implies that after teaching session you ask yourself how you think things went and what were your strengths/weaknesses, a kind of educational post-mortem assessment of how you think things went. For reflections-for-action you think about how you might do things differently the next time you do a similar session, based on your introspective analysis. Questions come up like 'Do I shorten the session?' 'Do I enhance parts and eliminate others?' This model always has me thinking about how to improve my teaching, in the moment after the session concludes and what I might do differently next time. It's a built-in quality control that only makes one better if we are honest.

- Lecturing is the best way to convey information. This is one of the biggest misnomers in medical education. There have been so many articles that have refuted this belief and yet the lecture is still the mainstay of how we convey information to trainees (Davis et al., 1999).

If one thinks about the process and model of lecturing, it represents a top-down approach to giving information to learners. It is usually a 'talk at participants', thereby not knowing if the learners are actually learning and not taking into account who the learners are. Let me be clear that presenting topics like results of cutting edge research or studies that impact patients or learners are likely best delivered by lecturing. For other subjects, it might be reasonable to consider models other than the teacher-talk only format. To activate learners in a traditional lecture context, one can use a couple of different models (Sarwary & Greenberg, 2019):

(1) Just-in-time teaching—This is a pedagogical model in which the lecturer uses feedback from learners in close proximity to the session. Although this was originally described for classroom teaching, it can be used in single sessions in medicine with the challenge being to encourage participants to complete the quiz before the session. Learners are sent these questions just before the session via iPhone or email and are asked to respond in a timely fashion. Not only does this model activate learners, it also provides faculty with information regarding how well or ill-prepared the learners are prior to the class, importantly identifying areas of difficulty affecting a large number of respondents. On the other hand, if the learners answer most of the questions correctly, the teacher can use class time for content at higher cognitive levels, such as application of knowledge in a clinical setting, rather than focusing on theory.

(2) Team-based learning (TBL)—This technique was developed 25 years ago to teach business principles. In this model, trainees again are activated in small groups in and outside the classroom, perhaps watching a video and reading a short assignment prior to class. In class they individually complete a 10-question quiz and then meet in their small groups to discuss answers to each of the questions, agreeing on the best answer for each question. In discussing answers in the reporting process, when groups disagree, the group that has correctly identified the correct answer teaches the group(s) that have not, explaining how they arrived at that answer. This is near peer teaching at its finest, with the faculty member watching this education unfold. In essence, this eliminates PowerPoint slides and decreases teacher talk to a minimum.

Again, most of classroom time is focused on higher order cognitive learning versus lower-level knowledge seen in lectures.

(3)  The flipped classroom (FC)—This parallels TBL but differs in that TBL is an ongoing process over a series of formal classroom time where the same groups stay together, not true of the FC. Also, there is no grading in this technique while there is in TBL. Lastly, this technique is an excellent format for including standardized patients and/or learners to help illustrate issues at higher cognitive levels; e.g., how to give bad news.

(4)  Interactive lecturing—The caveat using this technique is that the learner generally has an attention span of 15–20 min as a passive learner during a lecture (Steinert & Snell, 1999). Interjecting a case presentation, Hollywood or documentary film or provocative question at each 15–20-min period of the hour activates learners, refocuses the audience if their attention is straying, and sends the message that this session will require input from the participants (no time to sleep!!!). This model requires practice as time is limited and the teacher has to decide how much time to allow audience participation for each of the segments (at 15, 30 and 45 min). It's a balance between activating learners and providing important information. The other caveat is the one I mentioned above; i.e., I do not stand behind the podium which is a barrier between the speaker and the audience. In addition, teaching while walking is a principle I live by as it helps in getting the audience to follow and listen to you as you walk the lecture hall. Importantly eye contact is maintained as one walks, thereby engaging learners. I like to walk to the last row in the auditorium where medical students and residents hang out and engage them, suggesting I value them. When I request using a roving microphone to teach, it is my impression that this approach is an outlier in most if not all institutions. In summary, each of these four techniques allows the faculty member to be interactive with the group, incorporates high level cognition, and emphasizes the learner's responsibility for mastering the information at hand.

- Using learning objectives for a session that are at the bottom of Bloom's taxonomy. Many faculty are not familiar with this taxonomy, published in 1956. This is a hierarchical order cognitive taxonomy that was developed to help teachers in the classroom regarding content and evaluation. Using key verbs in the taxonomy for questioning, curricula development and formal lectures (like grand rounds) is important. At the bottom of the taxonomy are verbs which reflect knowledge and as one ascends the framework, the verbs become more action oriented, ultimately having the learner performing. Whereas knowledge is the basis for further learning, objectives for sessions should transcend knowledge. In the clinical arena, assessing knowledge is important when CEs interact with trainees, but once one has established that the trainee knows/does not know basic information, that can be the takeoff point to recognize what to teach. In the classroom or for a course, using verbs that assess higher cognitive learning in addition to knowledge is essential as they reflect how clinicians think and solve problems (e.g., Blooms: synthesize, analyze).

- Too many slides for a presentation and too much information on those slides. Since the lecture remains a major way faculty provide information, especially in grand rounds and for core sessions to colleagues and trainees, besides thinking about attention span and activating learners one should seriously consider (1) how much information is on each slide, (2) how many sides there are for each lecture, and (3) and how to use the slides as a prompt rather than reading them to the audience. Once I explored adult learning principles early in my career, I became at first consciously (and eventually unconsciously) aware of how faculty violate these principles. Having too much information on slides is a distraction for the audience as it is not unusual for the people to be reading the slides while the speaker is talking. Instead, there should be bullet points that contain key words describing where the speaker will be going with his next point(s). In addition, there are lectures where there might be 60 slides in a 50-min lecture. Trying to cover that many slides is close to impossible and requires the speaker to travel at 90 miles an hour, also not conducive to optimal learning. Bottom line is to reduce the number of slides (in my favorite grand rounds presentation, I use 32 slides that includes 4 movie clips) and the information on those slides to make your presentation more effective. As with most other educational models, more is not necessarily better.

- Answering learner's questions before he/she commits to the answer. I don't have references on this issue, but I know that the concept fits adult learning theory by activating the learner. It's not about what the teacher knows but rather how the trainee approaches the situation. When the trainees ask a question, there can be many reasons why. The trainee (1) may indeed not know the answer, (2) is looking for confirmation of his thoughts on the question, or (3) is inquisitive and searching for new knowledge. I will address this issue in two scenarios, one in the ambulatory and the other in the inpatient setting. Whichever the reason the trainee is asking the question, the teacher should respond with something like 'That is an interesting question.....what do you think the answer is?' Occasionally, a brazen trainee will reply that if she knew the answer, she wouldn't be asking the question. That is a rare occurrence, in my experience. In a group inpatient setting, once the trainee responds, it is ideal to ask the others in the group what they are thinking, again engaging as many learners as possible. That activates the learners besides the one asking the question and provides information to the teacher about the trainees' thinking on this patient. Acknowledging interesting thoughts is important as trainees always have perceptions and knowledge that can add to our being as a CE. Once everyone replies, the teacher can **then** state her thought processes on the question. In the ambulatory setting, a one-on-one situation, the response of the learner will dictate where the discussion goes. If the trainee states she has no idea what the answer is, I often segue into general disease categories, prompting the trainee to think about pathophysiology, stepping back to their basic science years. So, is this inflammatory, genetic, oncologic, vascular, autoimmune, etc. Once the learner responds to that approach, further questioning can focus on more specific information about the patient. Of course, that approach also can be applied in the inpatient setting. Based on anecdotal observations, we don't make an attempt to know our learners.

- Although time is of the essence and we are all pressed for time because we multi-task in academic medicine, we need to make an effort to know our learners. The reasons are that this exercise helps to set a safe learning climate and we can understand what learners bring to the plate based on their rich experiences. We can obtain that information in orientation, mentoring and informal discussions when there are brief periods of downtime. Knowing that a medical student spent a number of years working as a physician assistant provides information to which the teacher can refer when dealing with patients. That individual likely had numerous rich experiences during that time period, many of which may be pertinent to patient care. Not knowing that this person has had previous patient experiences is a major mistake and that information should govern the way we interact with that learner around patient care. Other trainees have had life experiences that impact how they think and approach medicine in general. An example is when a 4th year student thinking about surgery came to me as a possible mentor in pediatrics, I asked why she was thinking of changing specialties at this late date. In addition, I asked her to tell me something about herself that would be relevant. She offered that when she was 13 years of age, her older sister was involved in an auto accident that left her quadriplegic. Coming from a single parent family, this student decided herself to drop out of school and care for her sister, never asking her mother if this was ok. She eventually received a GED for high school, went onto college and the rest is history as she was accepted to medical school. How is that for resilience! To not know that information about a student is missing critical information on how people cope with adversity and succeed. Of course, there are so many other stories that help to shape trainees' professional and personal lives and the only way we know those is to ask. Besides trainees sharing with us, it is ok that we also share things about ourselves that helped shape our careers and lives. This is the beauty of a safe learning climate and a pathway deviating from the hierarchy of which most of us have been players. It's all about connections, trust, empowerment and humanism.
- Not thinking about levels of questions one uses with learners. In my observations of teaching on rounds and one-on-one in the ambulatory setting, it has been my experience that more often than not teachers exclusively use low level questions to query learners (Bloom, 1956). These questions require very little thinking as they basically pertain to knowledge one has acquired and not beyond. Trainee responses to these questions are very brief and do not involve any problem-solving or higher order thinking. These kinds of questions are necessary initially to assess the learner's knowledge and once the teacher determines through lower-level questioning that the learner has significant knowledge about a topic and patient problem, asking higher level questions on the taxonomy is important (the flipped classroom precludes having to use low -level questions in class and goes right to higher order thinking). As one ascends the cognitive functioning on Bloom's taxonomy, the complexity of thought processes gets increasingly

greater and requires the learner to think about synthesizing, analyzing and evaluating information. Mezirow in his work on transformative learning lists types of question like 'How', What, Why.' The 'what' questions are content-oriented, the 'how' process-oriented and the 'why' premise-oriented. Through these questions, faculty can assess how well the trainee problem-solves around a patient problem. Importantly, higher order thinking is really the way faculty solves patient problems!

- Not verbally addressing the competencies and milestones with trainees. In my short tenure seeing patients and precepting trainees in the era of competencies and milestones, I have observed anecdotally that neither residents nor medical students seem to know and be able to analyze the ACGME competencies and milestones project as these apply with each patient. In essence, I feel this is the responsibility of faculty leadership to initially discuss this process with residents at the start of each academic year and with students on each rotation, followed by faculty addressing these competencies and milestones with each patient interaction. There appears to be a need for a faculty development (FD) program to teach faculty how to engage trainees around these skills, which when discussed with trainees, should require minimal additional time involvement. As an example, I have asked trainees 'so what competency(ies) does this interaction with the patient represent?' Not uncommonly, those are straightforward, such as doctor-patient communication, systems-based practice, etc. Bottom line: Requiring trainees to understand and be able to identify the competencies and milestones (how they are progressing on a particular milestone) in general and with each patient is a way they take responsibility for their learning and not delegating this solely to faculty. It also activates them in the process and their keeping track of the competencies and milestones in a log is certainly reasonable as they traverse their education. The competency project is an investment incorporating the trainee and faculty, assuring the public, accrediting agencies, the training programs and the appropriate governing bodies that we are graduating competent future physicians.

- Not documenting your teaching effectiveness. This is one of the most important misconceptions in that not documenting what one does teaching-wise is a problem, especially when it comes to considering clinician educators for promotion. When I am asked to review faculty curricula vitae in my own institution and nationally, there is a major omission most of the time how one's teaching has impacted learners, only listing what teaching the faculty member did. A list of teaching experiences does not address quality and without that, there can be little said about how teaching contributes to one's promotion. So, as part of an educator portfolio, I am suggesting not only listing educational endeavors, but documenting those in your educator portfolio. I have suggested Brookfield's Critical Incident Questionnaire earlier in the book but there are certainly other ways to document how effective your teaching was. Even 'handcrafted' evaluation instruments can be useful, and I suggest you research the literature on teaching evaluations and select from those instruments rather than creating something de-novo. Of course, if you pilot your 'new' instrument with a group of trainees and make any changes based on their feedback, this can eventually be used in any educational scholarship project over time (see my previous reference from Teach Learn Med 2020). What your goal should be is for trainees to report in short narratives how your teaching might have impacted them; i.e., Do they plan to change their behavior based on your session? Have you impacted their knowledge base and if so, how do they see this translating into behavior change? Have you changed their thinking about a specific issue and if so, how? Based on your teaching as one criteria, did they select your specialty as a career choice? What I am suggesting is challenging the clinician educator to be more specific about detailing educational activities, specifically in this context, teaching, so that any internal or external reviewer can assess the value of that person to the institution and how that aligns with promotion.

- Being a content expert and effective teacher go hand-in-hand. I am struck by faculty who have expertise in a specific area and they perceive that this makes them an excellent teacher. When I generically address this issue, I point out that my wife majored in education and spent four years learning to be a teacher, with some practice opportunities. How is it that when we graduate from medical school, residency training or health science programs that we are automatically afforded the title of 'teacher' when many of us have had not teacher training? I always respect content expertise but have concerns about faculty who view faculty development programs/training as unnecessary because their content expertise trumps teacher training. I often wonder if there is some anxiety about how effective their teaching is when we examine that under the microscope. I reflect back on when I was told I was a great teacher early in my career and for whatever reason, questioned this perception of me. I knew I was very knowledgeable and well-read, quoting references every time I saw a patient with trainees. I also thought my interpersonal skills allowed me to connect with trainees. However, when I participated in my first faculty development program in the mid-70s, I realized I was not a great teacher but a great information-giver. I had no idea about learning theory and how trainees learn. I would suggest that this is also true of many of our faculty who don't see the need to participate in FD programs to become better teachers. Bottom line-There is no correlation with being a content expert and a great teacher IF there has not been some understanding and application of educational theory and adult learning principles, a robust literature in medicine. The key for busy faculty is to find some balance between reading about their clinical specialty and learning educational principles to enable them to be more informed teachers. Workshops, self-help books like this, being mentored and/or coached, peer-peer interactions, and short articles summarizing educational topics can help faculty attain this balance. The British Medical Journal had a series called Learning in Practice a number of years ago that had wonderful short articles on key topics like adult learning principles and feedback.
- Avoid saying 'I don't know'. This is a powerful statement from faculty to trainees and differs from saying that with patients (to be addressed under patient discussion). This statement conveys a humanistic aspect of faculty and provides the message that there is much uncertainty in medicine and healthcare and it is ok to say 'I don't know'. This messaging also conveys a safe learning climate and helps

to connect trainees with faculty. That is not the endpoint, however, in that when we don't know a diagnosis or information about a patient, it is incumbent for the team and faculty member to pursue this and figure out the most likely reason(s) for the patient's problems. It is not uncommon for trainees to offer a diagnosis and/or treatment plan no one else has considered, making a wonderful contribution to patient care and as a team member. It is interesting that some residents are uncomfortable when students pursue and find information important to patient care, i.e., not confident in their own identity. In the traditional hierarchy of each team, students are viewed at 'the bottom', but we have all seen individuals at that level shine when faculty and residents are stymied! This should be a welcomed part of the team in that all can contribute.

- Not thinking outside your comfort zone regarding teaching. My entire career can be characterized as looking for new adventures and not accepting the status quo. It implies risk-taking and working out of one's comfort zone. Going down new paths can also impact those around you and ideally you want to walk that path with others versus by yourself. One of the examples among many I can recall is after reading the Association for American Medical Colleges white paper entitled 'The General Professional Educational of the Physician' or GPEP Report (1981), I noted a section that addressed lecturing, basically stating that there was literally no information documenting behavior change after lectures. So, I reflected on whether or not we should keep lectures in the Pediatric clerkship that I headed. I decided to present this information to the clerkship committee, made up of many faculty that oversaw student education in their specialties in addition to medical student representatives. The group went along with the recommendation that we stop lectures in the clerkship, even though the students commented that these were the best quality lectures at the medical school in their clinical years. To insure a seamless transition from a lecture to an interactive model, I extended the session from one hour to 90 minutes and developed a FD program to teach faculty how to do interactive, case-based lecturing in that new timeframe. When I left my position as clerkship director, this model was still an integral part of student learning and always received rave reviews. In fact, on occasion when faculty reverted back to traditional lecturing, the students made negative comments about this deviation from the process. This all connects with the book Who Moved My Cheese: An Amazing Way to Deal With Change in Your Work and Your Life Spencer Johnson, G. P. Putnam's Sons 1998, 1st Edition in which the author, using an analogy of a colony of mice who have been living off an old and moldy piece of cheese. A couple of the mice (that could be you!) are concerned that there is something better cheese-wise outside their colony that they should explore. Most of the mice were concerned that risk-taking to finding new and better cheese was not worthwhile as why argue with what you have access to without any downsides? This analogy is poignant and implies that in order to be successful, creative and innovative, you have to think outside the box and take risks. These ventures do not always lead to successes; however we measure those. Understanding that not finding new sources of cheese the first time or couple of times is the risk you have to accept. However, finding a new source of food that is fresh and not moldy can be very rewarding for you and your colleagues. So, what cheese will you seek: moldy and diminishing in quantity or new and fresh?

- There is no need to teach communication skills to trainees post-medical school. Assuming that medical students remember everything they learned about effective communication skills in their medical school training is really a big assumption. They also had somewhat limited opportunities to apply some of the important principles about communicating with patients versus during residency training. Our residency training program at Children's recruits medical students from all over the country and my observations are that they all indeed need further teaching about communication skills. I am not certain if what I see are gaps in their training or whether or not they need reinforcing of these skills. Either way, it is not important what the underlying reason(s) are for these gaps. We just have to observe them to define what they do well and what they need to improve. In a couple of publications, I have addressed how residents give bad news, how they obtain information on the main concerns of parents and why that concerns them, and deciphering when a patient needs referral for a potential cardiac problem and how to counsel the patient appropriately (Carter Guice et al., 2021; Greenberg et al., 1999; Harasheh et al., 2016). In addition, I have worked with anesthesiology and Ob-Gyn residents about their communication skills and our research has shown short-term improvement with interventions. We have utilized standardized patients for practice opportunities in these situations, and trainees have appreciated the opportunities to interact with simulated patients to apply their new knowledge to actual patient care (Berger et al., 2010). All medical centers in North America have standardized patient programs and if these centers are like those at GWU, incorporating SPs into teaching and evaluation is certainly an option as one designs studies and curricula amenable to this methodology.
- Faculty know how to teach a skill. Whereas this may be true in some cases, this is another area where a faculty development offering can enhance knowledge and skills of faculty. There are so many instances where skill training is important, like teaching how to tie surgical knots, activating learners when they enter a room with faculty, teaching aspects of physical diagnosis, putting in a chest tube, and other skills. There are principles in teaching a skill, many of which are incorporated into adult learning theory. After discussing general aspects of skills teaching, facilitators will analyze and separate the skill into parts (see Bloom's taxonomy), model the skill, allow practice, and provide supervision of the skill through evaluation. All of these parts are essential in the process and recalibrating when the learner is having problems performing the skill is critical. An example here is taking a trainee into a patient room to demonstrate a skill, like a physical exam exercise or a communication skill. First, you and trainee need to agree on what the focus of this teaching session should be. Trainees are savvy about what they have not had observed and/or what their weaknesses might be. Once the focus is decided, faculty need to be specific on what will go on in the room and what the trainee needs to look for. As an example, if the focus is on percussing the abdomen, faculty might want the trainee to demonstrate first how she percusses, providing feedback when she's done. Having the trainee talk out loud on how

she is performing the procedure is helpful. If there is corrective feedback on this, the faculty attending will alert the trainee to watch how his hands are placed to percuss, perhaps talking out loud as the exam progresses. 'Look at the way I hold my hands and position my fingers to percuss. How did that compare to the way you did it'? Then, the dyad exits the room and there is a brief summary of what happened and what was learned. In this example, it is 180 degrees from saying to the trainee, 'Come into the room while I demonstrate how to do percussion.' The learner in this case enters the room without a clear sense of what is going to happen and is a passive bystander. Activating the learner (this technique is known as activated demonstration) is an adult learning principle and involves the learner in the process, assuring that effective learning is more likely to occur and this will hopefully translate into behavior change.

- Most residents don't need their counseling skills observed. In my experience at one institution, I have found that residents are rarely observed counseling patients. For me, it was a wonderful opportunity to observe them with their consent and see how they counseled patients over time. Uniformly (and I attribute this to no formal teaching in this area) they counseled patients top-down, with little input from and interaction with the patients/families. Whereas their counseling content was appropriate, they do not use skills to activate patients or families as part of a collaborative process. As an example, there are areas to consider that help to make patients/families partners in the interactions we have. Asking 'How will you explain the diagnosis and plan to a spouse/significant other/parent at home?' This verifies the patient understood what you said and is able to transfer that information accurately to someone else. Another question is 'Is there anything I have said that you are unable or not willing to do?' There might be barriers that preclude him for carrying out your instructions. Some or all of these might be surmountable once the patient discusses these with you. You also can ask how the patient pays for prescriptions as not having insurance can result in costs way beyond the patient's ability to pay. Even with insurance, some drugs are prohibitively expensive, and physicians do not always know prices and what insurance covers. Advice about non-prescription drugs can also be helpful as generic brands can be much less costly than name brands. However, patients need to be assured that generic drugs can be just as effective as name brands as they sometimes wonder if there are qualitative differences. Over-the-counter drugs are very expensive (how about $26 for 3 cc of eye hydration drops or $30 for a cough suppressant?) and can also be a barrier for some patients on adhering to medical advice. The key here is that effective counseling is interactive and not top-down. Observing trainees and providing feedback can change this model from top-down to interactive.
- Not teaching physicians the importance of silence in teaching/learning interactions. What am I talking about when I say 'silence'? I am speaking about 10–15 seconds where there is no talking. That period of time where there is silence can be very uncomfortable (try it…. mark off 15 seconds on your watch and see what I am speaking about). Whereas I will address silence during patient interviews, silence in teaching is also very important. I perceive this is difficult for faculty but silence often indicates one of three issues for the learner; namely,

she is sorting through information at higher cognitive levels to get the answer, the learner doesn't know the answer, or doesn't understand the question. In the first instance, this happens when the faculty member asks higher level cognitive questions on Bloom's taxonomy and those require deeper thinking and time to produce the results of the learner's thinking. That will be manifested in silence by the learner. With the second example, once the teacher establishes that the learner does not know the answer, rephrasing the question or using a different context (the pathophysiologic approach I mentioned earlier) can be helpful to the learner and can often lead to the correct answer. In the third example, asking the learner if the question was clear and again, try to reframe the question, based on the learner's uncertainty. Bottom line: Silence in teaching has some root causes and in general often means a reset in terms of reframing the question or waiting until the learner thinks through the problem.

- Not recognizing teachable moments, especially in the context of patient care. Teaching moments or critical incidents are seen frequently in the clinical setting and it is not predictable when they occur. This can be defined by questions that trainees ask, interest in specific comments you or others on the team make, or discussion about a patient that resonates with the teacher or the learner, what might be described as an 'aha moment'. It is easy to miss these opportunities as inpatient teams are on 'full steam ahead' mode as are interactions in the ambulatory setting. These moments take little time for the teacher to make a teaching point and then continue onto the responsibilities at hand. An example would be 'How does the presence or absence of splenomegaly affect your differential diagnosis in this patient?' This physical finding can be the difference between one diagnosis and another. Once the learner answers the question, the faculty member can make the teaching point that might be so important regarding patient care. Other examples, and there are more than anyone can count, could include Hoagland's sign in the presence of sore throat and lymphadenopathy seen in infectious mononucleosis and identifying a fixed split-second heart sound in a preschooler with a murmur. These are issues to which the learner has never been likely exposed and the teaching points here are quick and contextual.

- 'I don't know enough because I'm a junior clinician educator (CE) and that makes me feel inadequate'. Well, everyone starts at the junior level and we all make that eventual transition to mid-level and senior clinician educator. Your teaching job, as junior CE, is to be a great facilitator of learning. You don't have to have all the information at your fingertips but be a persistent learner yourself and read everything you can, especially about your patients. There will be plenty of times where you will not know information, but you and team can go forward and seek what information is missing. Don't feel like you have to be the 'sage on the stage' all the time. Involve your learners and get their input on different issues. Many of your trainees will have had interesting life experiences that could impact patient care and they need to share those if you give them that option. Also, as a junior CE, you can always seek opinions from more senior faculty when you are unsure how to proceed. Bottom line-you don't need to have all the knowledge expected of a more senior CE. Just be consistent with your teaching AND feedback and read. There should be some comfort for you to know that you will have had more experience than MOST of your trainees. Engage your trainees, help bring meaning to their work, bring enthusiasm to each interaction. Trainees appreciate that sincerity and commitment to their training.

- Teaching in the presence of the patient is generally not advisable. In the current environment there are many reasons why one would want to teach in the presence of the patient: (1) It saves time in the long-run, (2) It demonstrates connectedness of the team to the patient in the inpatient and the caregiver and patient in the ambulatory setting. (3) The patient gets an opportunity to hear the doctor(s) and trainee(s) discuss her problem, reinforcing that the CE and/or team are invested in the patient. There should be some ground rules on how the team functions in the presence of the patient. The patient/parents need to know when it is appropriate for their input and if it is ok to counter an issue they perceive as incorrect. This validates the patient as teacher and active part of the interaction.

  The downsides are that when the patient problem is a sensitive one regarding the diagnosis or treatment, it is better to discuss that outside the room initially (e.g., cancer, sexually-transmitted disease and life-altering diagnoses). Also, there is a need to return to the patient to further explain issues that occur during the discussion as these interactions can be quick and things the patient/family hear can be confusing. There can be a number of issues the patient did not understand and need clarification. With assistance from the faculty, a trainee can do that or the attending physician/healthcare provider can be the point person. Making certain the patient understood the conversation and nuances of what the team discussed is important. So, instead of telling the patient what occurred, the point person should ask the patient for his/her understanding of the conversation.

- Not having colleagues observe your teaching. This is important to do periodically if we are to grow and profit from timely feedback. In the *Primer* published in July, 2022, I relate a story about being observed twice by an internationally known medical educator and friend, Dr. David Irby. He provided feedback after the first workshop, and then he likely wanted to know how I used his feedback when facilitating the second workshop. This is a great example of peer observation of teaching. I mention a parallel model for patient care and would argue that (1) This doesn't happen often enough, if at all, (2) Having a colleague observe your teaching and provide you feedback is a great way to enhance and/or strengthen your teaching skills. (3) One can use the information obtained when observed in an educator portfolio, documenting your personal growth, and (4) What goes around, comes around: You should be observing colleagues teaching just as they observe you. In essence, these observations need not be prolonged and can be modeled after how we observe trainees. Observing in 5–15 min segments can result in important feedback on how we teach (Baumgartner et al., 2021). Actually, observing for 5 min intervals over time can provide a wealth of information about a faculty member's teaching. This observation model can enhance teaching in any academic center and highlights to others the educational priorities of the institution.

- Not negotiating what you want trainees to call you and vice versa. This issue is likely controversial and generational. Many healthcare providers like to be called doctor by trainees and that is based on a long tradition. I personally have viewed this as an area that can reinforce a safe learning climate and have negotiated this with trainees. My negotiation with trainees is to start with 'What should we call each other?' Invariably, trainees suggest 'Dr. Greenberg' and I respond with then 'I must call you Mr./Ms./They'. I suggest they find another alternative and this usually ends up in 'Dr. Larrie', which to me narrows the gap between trainees and myself versus the more formal 'Dr. Greenberg.' As an aside, I have been informed by healthcare professionals from the Caribbean that they always address physicians by doctor and the last name. They would never consider calling a physician by her first name, obviously a cultural tradition. On the other hand, it is very important for faculty to know the names of trainees on any rotation.
- When you see something, say something. I know this is a slogan from Homeland Security, but it also works in medicine. In academic medicine we see so many interesting patients with PE findings that can inform other colleagues and trainees. What may be relatively routine for you can be a major learning experience for others. Using the technique I have mentioned as activated demonstration, ask the patient's permission to have others (e.g., trainees, fellow faculty) enter the room and observe and/or exam the patient, and then invite trainees and colleagues to come to the exam room, prepping them for what they are about to see. Seasoned physicians might take for granted about interesting findings that might be commonplace for them but perhaps very new for trainees. An example might be reducing a nursemaid's elbow in pediatrics from a dislocation of the radius proximally. Having a patient in pediatrics with a retracted testis versus an undescended testis is another common finding that makes for a great teaching point. Another example is after observors see and describe a rash, pointing out the defining features of the rash (e.g., Pityriasis rosea) and differentiating it from other papulosquamous rashes can be an important teaching point for junior trainees. It is important to recognize that the mundane for more experienced physicians can be new and exciting for junior learners!!
- Not always enjoying our efforts and including meaning in our work. Whereas we often see ill patients and that makes it difficult to appreciate full enjoyment of our work, as teachers we should be instilling that our work is meaningful and we should be approaching it with a positive attitude. Of course, the politics in an institution where there are many involved is always a factor, but those issues should be the small minority of situations or perhaps we should be seeking employment elsewhere. Bringing meaning to medicine implies that we are here for more than the science, but also our altruistic, compassionate, ethical and humanistic ideals that shape the kinds of people we are. This is often the reason people are attracted to medicine and we should model these virtues for our trainees. These attitudes can be reflected in our teaching, showing enthusiasm, humor, collegiality, empathy, humanism, and connectedness to our trainees and patients. After all, teaching is often the reason many CEs have entered academic medicine, as physicians and health science professionals.

- Not being observant of the learner's needs. An example that always stands out in my mind was when I was co-conducting a workshop for neurosurgery residents, the session was delayed because the chief resident was engaged in surgery. When I started the session somewhat after the appointed time, those in attendance were demonstrating negative body language and obviously had concerns about starting this workshop late. I did not pick up on those messages and my colleague, who was facilitating the session with me, called timeout and assured the residents we would be cutting the workshop content so that they would leave on-time as scheduled. Following that recognition of learner needs, there seemed to be a release of tension and the interaction with those residents improved. Had I continued the workshop without recognizing learner needs, I am certain there would have been minimal learning. Just as we do with patients, we should be in-tune with our learners and make certain that our teaching is not just about our agendas. We should be consciously aware that students who declare their career choice early and are traversing the clerkship as a requirement can be engaged if we know their interests that might overlap with our specialty. The same can be said of residents who might be interested in a subspecialty but can learn a lot within general medicine. It is beneficial for both the teacher and learner to understand the learner's needs for that particular rotation, and as I have mentioned previously, that can be done with a learning contract and or simply having learners express their goals in an orientation.
- Not making teaching contextual. Ideally, we teach around patient problems and the content overlaps with their diagnosis and treatment. On occasion, I have heard trainee complaints that the teacher focuses more on his favorite research topic rather than issues specific to the patient. Or the depth of the discussion around a patient problem can be more than any of the trainees need to know. Of course, discussions about the patient that are not focused or contextual can be distractions for trainees and perceived as not important regarding their learning. This approach also distances the learner and may make him seem uninterested. Adult learning theory emphasizes how learners become more involved when they see the learning as contextual and patient-related.
- Not analyzing and addressing why a trainee seems unengaged. When a trainee appears uninterested or unengaged in content in a specific rotation, in my experience there are six major reasons: (1) the goals and objectives of the rotation are either not stated or unclear, (2) trainees are not activated or significantly involved in the daily routine for that rotation, whether it may be patient care or education, (3) faculty do not make their teaching contextual, connecting patient care with learning, (4) roles, responsibilities and expectations are not explicit, (5) the learner has a medical or educational problem that has not been previously discussed with faculty, such as a learning disorder, and (6) for specific instances, the learner's learning preferences can be out-of-synch apropos to how she is being taught. Learners tend to 'drift' and seem uninterested when they are not certain of what is expected of them. Whereas they may learn specific material in a self-directed way, they may appear indifferent with faculty. These issues can generally be precluded by providing trainees with an orientation; emphasizing to faculty to

activate learners during the rotation; and talking to learners when you sense they are not 'in-synch' with you, making certain they are medically ok. An example that was so poignant was when an affable and very respected division head at GWU approached me and said the fellows in his department were feeling left out and ignored, especially at their weekly conference when current patients on the service were presented. I asked if I could attend an upcoming conference and upon entering the room, I noted a long table with chairs in the center and then single chairs ringing the perimeter of the room. As faculty and trainees filed in, all the seats at the table were taken by faculty, with fellows, residents and medical students assuming the single chairs on the perimeter. Watching teacher versus learner talk, the faculty dominated the discussion and fellows were seldom engaged, except when someone presented the patient. Residents and students rotating on the service were not at all involved. When I presented my findings after two observations and asked the chair if what I was observing was typical, he responded affirmatively. The hierarchy in this situation was very obvious to an outside observer and the fellows indeed did have a justifiable complaint about their learning issues. The chair was very grateful and subsequently changed the way the seating occurred, with trainees mixed in with faculty. That impacted the dynamics of teaching and learning, and fellows were quite happy with the change and outcome. Again, a trainee seemingly being unengaged can be a warning sign for the CE that is either trainee or teacher-related. Having a peer observe how you teach might shed some light on the situation.

- Delegating teaching responsibilities is risky. Not true at all!! I have tasked students and residents to assume the teaching role by researching an area related to patient care and they always do a superb job. Whereas most of the teaching CEs do is spontaneous and not something for which we prepare, giving trainees an opportunity to present a short blurb (3–5 min) on a topic involving a patient allows them to contribute to and feel part of the team and activates them. This should be followed with feedback by the CE in a timely fashion. Again, it is not important that the CE takes responsibility for all the teaching for a rotation and delegating this to others is reasonable. As mentioned earlier, we are all learners and potentially all teachers. Role-modeling how we teach and allowing trainees to emulate our behavior in part or totally is how teaching excellence perpetuates itself.

- Teacher training is an option for CEs. I know I am biased, but I don't view the world this way. Whereas teacher training programs are more numerous in medical schools and residency programs today, there are still many faculty who are not trained how to teach. That is alarming because teaching is one of the CE's major responsibilities. I previously related that my wife went to school 4 years to become a teacher, and that included a student teaching experience for a semester (included lesson plans, reporting to an advisor, being observed) and faculty automatically are accorded this designation as teacher when they finish medical school. Scary, isn't it? Faculty development includes so many aspects of how we teach, interact with our learners and provide feedback. Workshops exist at medical centers, universities, national meetings and stand-alone conferences. Institutions can step up and make faculty development an integral part of the ongoing professional development of faculty. Those faculty who receive poor evaluations consistent over time should be removed from teaching trainees contingent on their participating in faculty development workshops or courses on teaching and learning. There have been instances in our school where faculty have been abusive to students and they have been removed from teaching responsibilities.

- The trainees have not prepared for a teaching session by reading an assigned short article. There are occasions when you ask trainees to read a short and pertinent article/chapter so as to engage them in interactive conversation around patient care. I am certain this approach I suggest will be debated by many, but I see two choices if they have not read the article and are not prepared for the teaching session: (1) carry on with the conference, with you taking the top-down lead, (2) cancel the conference. I have always chosen the 2d option when having had inpatient responsibilities (now assumed by hospitalists) as I consider this situation an example of non-professionalism. Let me make certain I frame this so one understands my position. Firstly, I would clearly state during an orientation about expectations regarding teaching and learning during the rotation; i.e., I am sharing those activities with trainees and expect them to assume responsibility for their learning. Secondly, any conferencing on the rotation would be very pertinent to patient care and hopefully contribute to trainees' knowledge and skills. Thirdly, expecting busy trainees who are at different levels on the learning curve to do extra reading can be overwhelming **if** the CE suggests an article that is beyond a few pages or 10–12 min to read. That being said, I have certain expectations of trainees as part of their professional growth and adhere to those values. I think my wife and I reared our children using the same principles by setting limits, being clear about our expectations, and allowing freedom in a balanced and parallel way as long as this happened within the limits. I have been known to voice my displeasure when trainees have not assumed responsibility for their learning and have cancelled a learning session based on that choice. There is nothing wrong with being a firm teacher when expectations are laid out very clearly and the learners have not held up their end. See any similarities to being a CE and parenting?

- Not fine-tuning our small group teaching skills. This is one of the most common teaching venues for CEs and participating in faculty development workshops addressing this topic should be value-added (Tiberius, 1999). Group dynamics are very different than one-on-one teaching, although many of the principles of adult learning theory apply here. It is not uncommon in a group for there to be unclear goals of a session, the learning environment might not feel 'right' (e.g., some trainees may feel they are 'on-the-spot'), uneven participation by trainees, and some of the trainees not asked to participate at all, the hierarchy to which I previously referred. Knowing how to troubleshoot these issues as a group facilitator is critical if one is to be an effective teacher who has a reputation for promoting learning. Small group teaching/learning can be in the form of the flipped classroom, just-in-time teaching, team-based or problem-based learning, or simply rounds and informal sessions. Faculty development in this area should provide content and process issues that come up when teaching in small groups.

As an example, when a trainee asks a question that doesn't seem pertinent to the discussion or makes a response that could be interpreted as 'off-base', how should the CE handle either of those?

- Not actively engaging learners in a poster presentation at a national, regional or local meeting. I mentioned this point in my Primer but this bears repeating. It actually transcends teaching and educational scholarship (ES) but the emphasis here is on process and not content. Poster sessions represent peer reviewed abstracts and have the potential to be the one of the most interactive educational opportunities (in addition to workshops), sometimes leading to future collaborations. These sessions can also be represented over many days of a conference and seemingly go on forever in large exhibit halls. There are a couple of factors that are real and underly why I push activating learners who are viewing the posters: (1) There are many posters for participants to view over what is a limited time period for any of them, (2) There is usually a significant amount of information on a poster to read, and (3) Participants might have limited time to see specific poster that interest them. Thus, I am suggesting a way to engage participants as to gleaning the most important points of your study. Although I have not seen published information on this topic, when participants stop momentarily to see my poster AND make eye contact with me, I immediately reach out and ask what their interests might be in the study and if I could summarize the highlights. This should be somewhat 'prepared' before the session as you do want to be succinct, respecting that person's time. In fact, there might be more than one person viewing the poster when this happens, meaning you might be summarizing for a couple of people at any one time. When this occurs, this grouping of people often attracts others out of curiosity, likely because they see a small 'crowd' and assume something interesting is happening. These interactions can lead to questions you might not have considered, rich discussions, interjection of someone else's ES that might be similar and suggestions for the next iteration of the study. It also is an opportunity to meet new colleagues with like interests in ES and ongoing communication. Some of the more concrete results such as evolving into a collaborative study can be entered into one's educator portfolio (EP). If indeed you know that your presentation encouraged a colleague to pursue aspects of your study, this also can be included in your educator portfolio (EP) as way to demonstrate your teaching effectiveness.

- Assumptions about what learners know regarding the H&P. Whereas medical students receive intensive training in performing a H&P in their first 18 months of medical school, they lack experience in this area and the CE should not assume they are competent. Residents have historically received even less attention to their communication and physical diagnosis skills. Going over their findings early on is important until one recognizes they have achieved milestones in this area. It is through these repetitive iterations with supervision that trainees learn to do an excellent H&P. Focusing on specific areas over time (chest, heart, abdomen) with trainees can help them master these small chunks of learning more easily. As an example, I have precepted many residents over time who have presented a patient whom they state has a heart murmur. What sometimes is missing from this presentation is the character of that murmur on physical exam; i.e., the second heart sound and how it is split, the femoral pulses (in the pediatric age group), where the murmur is loudest over the precordium, the cardiac rhythm, and characterization of the precordium on palpation. The absent of this information does not allow an accurate assessment of whether or not the patient has cardiac pathology or not. I am concerned, coming from another generation, that trainees are learning, through modeling by residents and yes, faculty, that the physical exam is subservient to imaging studies that define the problem. This is another example of why the US spends so much on medical care compared to other nations, with patient outcomes not necessarily improved. I have previously mentioned how observation of H&P skills can enlighten faculty about what trainees do well and what they can improve.

- Language doesn't matter when engaging learners. Actually, language is everything when we speak with patients (parents) and learners. Sometimes, unconsciously (or even worse, consciously), we might use language that is demeaning to those in the hierarchy that are at the lowest rungs on the ladder. A common example would be 'You know this information about x disease, correct?' This is a question making an assumption about what one thinks a learner should know. I have addressed this issue in the point about learning climate. Part of that implies a connection between learners and faculty, meaning that there is mutual respect that has to be earned in addition to a trusting relationship. In reality, learners would be free to say to a CE in a feedback session that he/she felt demeaned by a statement made on rounds, as an example. In fact, what occurred might not have been a demeaning comment but constructive criticism about a patient care issue. However, as my wonderful wife of 60 years will attest, it's not always the content that's the issue but the tone of the conversation. This tone can also subliminally reflect biases that have infiltrated one's persona. Being in-tune from whence one has come is critical in the tone and type of language CEs use with trainees. Every one of us has been at lower end of the rung. Let's not forget that as we ascend the hierarchical ladder. Let's use language in our teaching that promotes collaboration, respect and caring.

- Not advocating for our learners. Again, another part of a safe learning climate is to have CEs advocating for learners. The hierarchy we have inherited in Western medicine has not gone away and our trainees are at the bottom of the rung on the ladder. They need our input on issues they might see as problems and to be there to listen to them and hear their concerns. That does not mean we always have to agree with them, but availing ourselves to convey that we care and are willing to listen is important in these chaotic days of national policy changes, top-down decisions without all the stakeholders' comments, diversity and inclusion issues, access to medical care problems, and other emotionally-laden topics. Today's generation often see themselves as advocates for the disenfranchised and see that social fabric as intertwined with their education and relationship to patients. Hearing our trainees incorporate social medicine into their problem-solving and trying to understand healthcare disparities is very important as is supporting their passion when appropriate. The generational differences between our trainees and CEs can be significant and may make it difficult to understand some of their values as compared to ours (e.g.; work ethic, pay, work hours, commitment to patient care). Best advice is to be a good listener and try to understand their points of view. Once we comprehend their stance on an issue, like career choice, we can better advise and counsel them regarding this context.

- Expressing negative and perhaps demeaning emotions and body language when the learner states 'I don't know the answer to that question', especially after you have previously taught the learner that topic. I also mention this same scenario in response in patient care, and in a parallel fashion the learner has not comprehended what you have taught. I previously mentioned Jerry Harvey's name (Professor Emeritus, School of Management, GWU; deceased) who cleverly and poignantly said that he knew when he was teaching, but he didn't always know when learners were learning. In fact, we might well have 'taught' the learner something about a specific patient but there are times when the learner 'doesn't get it'; i.e., hasn't learned what we have taught. When this same teaching point arises again with a similar patient and the learner acts as if this was the first-time hearing this, we as teachers might be inappropriately angry about an issue we have previously taught. In fact, we have not done our job; i.e., we have not determined if and what the learner has learned and hopefully applied to patient care. Simply asking learners after making a teaching point what the 'take-home message' is helps to validate that they have learned what you have taught, or not! Assuming learners are at fault when they don't comprehend a topic we taught hearkens back to the old hierarchy of the teacher is the supreme one and invincible.
- Inviting trainees to see an interesting finding on a patient without preparing them. There are always interesting findings on physical exam with patients and having trainees see patients with those findings is important for their growth. To facilitate the interaction, the following should be considered: First of all, the patient has to give permission for others to come into the room. Once that is done, the faculty member then alerts the group or individual as to what they will be seeing. This model is called activated demonstration. A physical finding you might want trainees to learn is in a patient with cystic fibrosis who has chronic obstructive pulmonary disease and is sitting forward in bed with tachypnea. Telling the group to watch from the door of the room and relate what they are seeing is a good teaching point and reinforces observation. It is not unusual for medical students to miss this teaching point, which then becomes the focus of a brief discussion of the importance of observation. Another example is the importance of examining the abdomen of a patient who has a large spleen, identifiable by starting palpation at the iliac crest, moving cephalad, and then using percussion to determine it's size. Bottom line: Prepare the trainee(s) for what you want them to do/see as your teaching point.
- In the 1970s, as a junior CE I was told I was an excellent teacher. Not knowing if this was an accurate description, I attended my first faculty development conference over a three-day period. Leaving that session, I realized that I was a great information-giver, not an excellent teacher. I was not aware at the time of adult learning theory and how that impacts how we teach. That conference set the tone for my career in education, as my interest was piqued in defining excellence in education. My advice to junior CEs is to find faculty development programs in

one's own school, national meetings, online opportunities (master's degrees), and through mentoring with faculty who are well-versed in educational principles. I am not advocating for all faculty to make education the focus one's career but using education as a vehicle for teaching one's specialty.

- Not recognizing the dynamics between the teacher and learner. Gerald Grow has developed a model for how learners and teachers interact, realizing there are learners who are very self-directed and others who are teacher-dependent (Grow, 1991). Likewise, there are teachers who are very facilitative and those who are authoritarian. Grow addresses where there are matches and mismatches between teachers and learners, which can often explain how effectively trainees learn. These similarities and differences can help explain when learners are mastering information in your presence and when there are obvious learning difficulties because of mismatches. Recognizing learning styles and preferences was one of the early principles I learned from Agnes Rezler, a superb education from the University of Illinois, former Center for Medical Education. It enabled me to understand how I learn best depending on the context of the situation, sometimes independently, other times in groups; sometimes concretely, other situations abstractly.

- Performance is not necessary to be an excellent teacher. I have found many faculty are not familiar with the Dr. Fox experiment (Ware & Williams, 1975) in which an actor lectured to a group of mental health professionals on a topic on which they would likely have little knowledge. Lecturing in an animated and enthusiastic manner without attention to content was rated highly by those health professionals, meaning they seemed to value process over content. This experiment has been reproduced a number of times with the same outcome: Teacher personality trumps content! My assessment of this now 50-year-old study is that faculty must have a blend of knowledge about a topic mixed with enthusiasm, passion, humor and other characteristics that would help engage learners.

- Not citing seminal studies, stories and history in your teaching. There are certainly many important tidbits of information that can be a perspective on what one teaches that can inform learners about from whence we come. I have found a paucity of pediatricians knowing the seminal studies of Barbra Korsch in the 60s about communication skills, many of which are the basis of effective communication with patients today (Korsch et al., 1968). Trainees and junior faculty often do not seem to recognize our past in medicine and take-for-granted what we have in the present. Another example is the MRI for imaging in patients. This technique was studied by medical researchers and physicists in the US and Britain in the 70–80s and first applied to medicine in the late 70s, less than 50 years ago. Lastly, when I occasionally see a patient with EBV (aka, infectious mononucleosis) I speak about the little-known booklet written by General Hoagland, then commandant from West Point who writes about his amazing experience with this disease in cadets matriculating there. Hoagland's sign, periorbital edema in patients with EBV, is mentioned in that booklet. In summary, it is mandatory, in my opinion, that we recognize those in the past who have paved the way for better medical care and education today.

- Pimping or badgering trainees is one way to elicit knowledge from them. This technique, which seems to be a throwback to the English system, has never been shown to be effective in interactions with trainees and in my opinion, is a form of incivility in medicine. It certainly is not conducive to a trainee's development of self-esteem and confidence in medicine. I distinguish that from questioning in a caring manner to enable trainees to solve problems.
- Not developing a professional intimacy between CEs and trainees. It is important to define relationships between faculty and learners, sharing information with each other about traversing life's challenges along the continuum of medical education and how one balances professional and personal lives. This does not imply that these relationships will result in friendships or anything beyond the professional realm. However, allowing trainees to understand our own travels and how we got there can be very informative for trainees.

# References

Baumgartner, S., Agrawal, D., & Greenberg, L. (2021). The enhanced brief structured observation model: Efficiently assess trainee competence and provide feedback. *MedEdPORTAL, 5*(17), 11153. https://doi.org/10.15766/mep_2374-8265.11153. PMID: 34013022; PMCID: PMC8096882.

Berger, J. S., Blatt, B., McGrath, B., Greenberg, L., & Berrigan, M. J. (2010). Relationship express: A pilot program to teach Anaesthesiology residents communication skills. *Journal of Graduate Medical Education, 2*(4), 600–603. https://doi.org/10.4300/JGME-D-10-00012.1

Bloom, B. S. (1956). Taxonomy of educational objectives: the classification of educational goals. Longmans, Green.

Brookfield, S. D. (1995). *Becoming a critically reflective teacher*. Jossey-Bass.

Carter Guice, M. D., Kristine Schmitz, M. D., Annette Aldous, M. P. H., & Greenberg, L. (2021). Observing Paediatric residents' communication skills during sick visits: Do they determine caregivers' main concern and their reasons for concern and are caregivers satisfied? *AMSRJ, 7*, Spring.

Chokshi, B., Battista, A., Merkebu, J., Hansen, S., Blatt, B., & Lopreiato, J. (2023). The SOAP feedback training program. *The Clinical Teacher, 20*(6), e13611. https://doi.org/10.1111/tct. 13611

Davis, D., O'Brien, M. A., Freemantle, N., Wolf, F. M., Mazmanian, P., & Taylor-Vaisey, A. (1999). Impact of formal continuing medical education: Do conferences, workshops, rounds, and other traditional continuing education activities change physician behavior or health care outcomes? *JAMA, 282*(9), 867–874. https://doi.org/10.1001/jama.282.9.867. PMID: 10478694.

Farrell, T. S. (2013). Reflecting on ESL teacher expertise: A case study. *System, 41*(4), 1070–1082).

Greenberg, L. W. (2004). Medical students' perceptions of feedback in a busy ambulatory setting: A descriptive study using a clinical encounter card. *Southern Medical Journal, 97*(12), 1174–1178. https://doi.org/10.1097/01.SMJ.0000136228.20193.01. PMID: 15646753.

Greenberg, L. W., Ochsenschlager, D., O'Donnell, R., Mastruserio, J., & Cohen, G. J. (1999). Bad news: A paediatric department's evaluation of a simulated intervention. *Paediatrics, 103*(6), 1210–1217.

Greenberg, L. (2020). Can the recruitment of senior transitioning clinician educators enhance the number and quality of resident observations? Thinking outside the box. *Teaching and Learning in Medicine, 32*(5), 569–574. https://doi.org/10.1080/10401334.2020.1801442

Grow, G. O. (1991). Teaching learners to be self-directed. *Adult Education Quarterly, 41*, 125–149.

Harasheh, A. S., Ottolini, M., Lewis, K., Blatt, B., & Greenberg, L. (2016). An innovative pilot curriculum training Pediatric residents in referral and communication skills on a cardiology rotation. *Academic Pediatrics, 16*, 700–702.

Harvey, J. B. (1979). Learning to not teach. *Exchange: The Organizational Behavior Teaching Journal, 4*(2), 19–21. https://doi.org/10.1177/105256297900400205

Hewson, M. G., & Little, M. L. (1998). Giving feedback in medical education: Verification of recommended techniques. *Journal of General Internal Medicine, 13*(2), 111–116. https://doi.org/10.1046/j.1525-1497.1998.00027.x

Jewett, L., Greenberg, L., Foley, R., et al. (1985). 774 Another look at career choice and learning styles. *Pediatric Research, 19*, 239. https://doi.org/10.1203/00006450-198504000-00804

Korsch, B. M., Gozzi, E. K., & Francis, V. (1968). Gaps in doctor-patient communication. 1. Doctor-patient interaction and patient satisfaction. *Pediatrics, 42*(5), 855–871. PMID: 5685370.

Ottolini, M. C., Ozuah, P. O., Mirza, N., & Greenberg, L. W. (2010). Student perceptions of effectiveness of the eight step preceptor (ESP) model in the ambulatory setting. *Teaching and Learning in Medicine, 22*(2), 97–101. https://doi.org/10.1080/10401331003656454

Plack, M. M., & Greenberg, L. (2005). The reflective practitioner: Reaching for excellence in practice. *Pediatrics, 116*(6), 1546–1552. https://doi.org/10.1542/peds.2005-0209. PMID: 16322184.

Sarwary, M., & Greenberg, L. (2019). Review of three educational models that enhance student learning: Alternatives to lecturing. *American Medical Student Research Journal, 6*, 1–6.

Steinert, Y., & Snell, L. S. (1999). Interactive lecturing: Strategies for increasing participation in large group presentations. *Medical Teacher, 21*(1), 3742. https://doi.org/10.1080/0142159998011

Tiberius, R. G. (1999). *Small group teaching; A troubleshooting guide*. Routledge.

Ware, J. E. Jr., & Williams, R. G. (1975) The Dr. Fox effect: a study of lecturer effectiveness and ratings of instruction. *Journal of Medical Education, 50*(2), 149–156. PMID: 1120118.

# Chapter 3
# Patient Care

Patient care is the essence of why most of us entered medicine, with the minority of healthcare and health science professionals seeking to do research as their major focus. CEs provide the majority of patient care in academic settings, as both generalists and subspecialists. We utilize patient care as the nidus for teaching others how to communicate, ensuring trainees perform thorough and accurate Hx and PEs, arrive at appropriate diagnoses and treatment plans, and model for them ideal ways to take care of patients. We also generate ideas for research and educational scholarship from our patients and advocacy evolves from the problems with which our patients present. In today's revenue-driven environment, CEs, specifically in the ambulatory setting, are held to numbers of patients seen and how efficient they can be. They are asked to balance their patient care responsibilities with seeing those patients that initially interact with medical students, residents and health science trainees, making certain they provide quality teaching along the way. In the inpatient units, hospitalists oversee an array of seriously ill patients, again balancing their care with teaching our future physicians and health science professionals around these problems. The purpose of this section is not to address the standards of care for specific diseases but to provide some general principles that are inherent in providing patient care. Many of these issues overlap with and may be inseparable from administrative and teaching areas.

- The front desk and the personnel assisting you are not your concern as they report to a non-medical person administratively. How the patient is treated before ever seeing you can have a major impact on how that patient feels emotionally in the exam room. Having to wait excessive periods of time and not have someone inform the patient that the doctor or health science professional is running late because of patient emergencies or problems is a mistake. Treating every patient with respect and warmth when they enter our domain and continuing that throughout their visit is very important. The treating healthcare professional needs to be assured that personnel interacting with the patient before seeing him are welcoming, warm and courteous; i.e., front desk/registration and nursing personnel. Breaches of

L. Greenberg M. D., *Misadventures in Patient Care and Medical Education*, SpringerBriefs in Education, https://doi.org/10.1007/978-3-031-83930-6_3

this expected behavior need to be called out by whomever supervises people in these positions. Neutral or negative behaviors can have a detrimental effect on the patient before you ever see him. In synch with what I said when entering a patient room and seeing what appears to be an angry or upset patient needs to be addressed. The retort when you state that the patient looks angry/upset is often, 'You would be upset too if you had to wait an hour to be seen'. Once you know this, I find this situation can be defused almost 100% of the time by stating 'I am so sorry that you were not informed that I am running late. Your time is also valuable'. Whereas administrative and medical/health science professionals do not have the same oversight reporting, they are, in fact, a team and need to function seamlessly in order to for patients to feel welcomed and respected. Some years ago when a Fortune 500 consultant from GWU was visiting NASA and stopped to speak with someone from environmental services, he asked that person what he did at NASA. He replied proudly that he was part of the team sending a man to the moon. It's this kind of invested and integrated teamwork that makes a practice valued by patients.

- Not comfortable dealing with uncertainty. There is so much we don't know about medicine, even being in the middle of a technology and information explosion over the last two decades. The most important teaching point here is that performing a complete history (Hx) and physical exam (PE) leads to a diagnosis up to 90% of the time. I always prided myself on being an excellent communicator and performing a thorough and accurate physical exam. That said, there are still so many times when I did not know the exact diagnosis. Not knowing the diagnosis was not uncomfortable to me as I gained more experience in patient care. It also did not push me to do unnecessary tests to better define the diagnosis. I believe the keys to uncertainty are the following: (1) Be thorough, (2) Assessing the severity of illness of the patient and be clear in your thinking about likely diagnoses. I have seen children with 40-degree Celsius temperatures who are running around the exam room and do not look ill. On the other hand, some patients just do not look 'right' and their demeanor and appearance signal they are significantly ill. Those are the patients in which I pursue testing. (3) Make certain you imply that you are partners with the patient and caregiver, and need for her to communicate over time when things are not going well. (4) Follow-up is what is most critical here. I always say to the patient 'Tomorrow should be better than yesterday…if not so, I need to hear from you.' (5) In my long career in academic medicine, I found that the huge majority of illnesses resolved in a few days and the patient that did not improve was an outlier. So, what might look like uncertainty initially may well resolve itself or develop into something detectable, like a urinary tract infection or fever resolving and a rash evolving in a child (roseola), and (6) Involve fellow faculty in your practice as another assessment of your patient and also consider a referral to a subspecialist As healthcare professionals, we do not love uncertainty, but illnesses evolve even though the diagnosis may not be so evident early on. Just remember to be thorough and ensure good follow-up with your patients.
- The threat of malpractice suits should guide the way we practice. I practiced more than 46 years and never was involved in a malpractice suit in my career.

Maybe that was lucky as so many suits are frivolous and have no merit. That being said, I have always taught trainees to be personable and courteous with patients, even when the two sides are apart; and to be thorough in their Hx, PE and counseling skills, recording all pertinent information in the electronic medical record as necessary. An example is when you use an ophthalmoscope to examine the red reflex in a newborn's eyes, record that that reflex was present bilaterally versus noting that 'the PE was normal'. When one does the latter and a problem occurs later on (retinoblastoma, cataracts), it is unclear from the record if the exam was performed and recall of that exam later is not always accurate. Also, patients sometimes want us to do tests that are costly, taking technicians' valuable and limited time, and do not add value to the diagnosis and treatment plan. I have heard many times from parents 'Aren't you going to do something for my child?' That implies aren't you going to do testing. My answer to that pertinent question is 'I have done something: I did a complete Hx and PE on your child and have basically eliminated many diagnoses that are serious'. When conflicts are not resolvable through civil conversation, having a more senior faculty member intervene or calling a patient representative/ombudsman to speak with the parent/ patient is appropriate. In the large majority of cases, issues that arise where there is misunderstanding or confusion are resolved amiably. Bottom line: When you are thorough in your H&P and interactive and caring with the patient, **there is no need to practice defensive medicine**. This model is NOT insurance that there will not be a malpractice suit, but it does tend to hold up over time based on my experience with thousands of patients.

- Patients have a right to demand to have a more senior person caring for them as opposed to a trainee. In a teaching hospital where CEs work, it is within the informed consent document that this indeed is a teaching (academic) center and that the patient, by signing this document, agrees to have trainees involved in their care. Of course, who reads those long consent forms we all are asked to sign before receiving care? So, if this issue is unclear to the patient, it is incumbent for more senior staff to inform the patient and assure her that there will also be an attending physician/healthcare professional involved in her care. In addition, some patients incorrectly believe that residents are not physicians and they may ask why a doctor is not seeing them. Again, an explanation is warranted as patients do not always understand the hierarchy of medical training. More junior trainees require an attending physician/health science professional to see the patient physically and of course, that is also necessary for billing purposes. It is incumbent upon those caring for patients to delineate who they are and their position in the hierarchy. Residents need to emphasize they are physicians and report to a more senior physician. Medical students or health science students also are responsible for identifying who they are and their title. They can state they are not physicians or health science faculty and that a more senior member of the faculty will be seeing them. Some institutions require a name badge to identify the person and position. There can also be instances where a patient has preferences for gender or race for their physician, also not appropriate in an academic center situation. In instances like this, a more senior staff member should intervene in a non-confrontational way, explaining the ground rules inherent in the consent form. If that does not resolve the conflict, a patient navigator can interact with the patient, again affirming the procedures in the center. Lastly, patients need to know when making an appointment if a nurse practitioner or physician assistant will be providing care as opposed to the physician overseeing the practice. This is no way suggests that care will be altered as the physician of record always assumes ultimate responsibility for the care.

- Not being transparent about decision-making when considering a diagnosis and plan for the patient. A way to engender trust and an open relationship with a patient is to basically 'talk out loud' about what you are thinking regarding the patient's diagnosis and what tests you are considering to confirm or deny what you are thinking as the main diagnostic possibilities. This transparency should be in-synch with how the patient wants information conveyed; i.e., wants to know everything versus letting the healthcare professional do what is necessary without patient involvement, and then some point in-between these two opposite poles. Not understanding why certain tests are performed and their frequency can be confusing to the patient and suggests lack of collaboration in decision-making. The treating professional can state why he/she/they are looking for, making testing and the CE's thinking more transparent. With the ability of patients to access a portal and sometimes 'know' test results before the physician/health science professional can be difficult. Advising patients that one will discuss the test results over the phone or in-person is important, especially if the patient accesses the results before the physician or healthcare professional. I would think advising the patient not to access test results before the physician does is reasonable so as not to engender undue anxiety.
- Dismissing patients from your practice who do not adhere to medical advice. As an example, in Pediatrics, we have too many parents who refuse vaccines for their children, using incorrect data obtained from social media about vaccines and putting selfish needs ahead of the good of the public. It is easy just to dismiss these patients when they feel this way, especially if there is no change in their views after the healthcare professional provides them with true informed consent (decision-making). Some of their beliefs are from a religious point of view, others from fear that vaccines cause autism and other serious illnesses, and others are part of conspiracy theories advocated by anti-vaxers. Whatever the reason(s), it is important to continue to provide evidence-based information to these patients over time, winning their confidence, and hopefully changing their beliefs. That, in my opinion, is a far better path than saying to the patient that you cannot care for them if they behave this way. Being overtly affirmative, one can say to the patient that you do not agree with their approach but because you care, you will continue to work with them. Of course, this analogy can include issues such as obesity, smoking, non-adherence to taking necessary medications, etc. There can be many reasons why the patient doesn't adhere to medical advice, some of them being socioeconomic, environmental (if you live in a shelter, it is not easy to follow a healthcare professional's treatment plan), mental health issues, and lack of trust in the system. My bias is to stick with the patient and through supportive and

collaborative behavior, hope to sway the patient to take the evidence-based path. Of course, this decision to support the patient can change over time depending on the situation. Lastly, in an academic setting we likely have reduced ability to dismiss patients from our practice, although there may be instances where parting ways with the patient is mutual and referring a patient to our colleagues with their permission may be a possibility. Transferring a patient needs to be discussed with the patient and the reasons why in addition to documenting this carefully in the medical record.

- It is not common for patients to be physically and/or verbally abusive with health-care providers. Studies have shown an alarmingly high number of healthcare professionals who have experienced verbal abuse from patients and fewer but a significant number who have been attacked physically. Some of this may be gender related, although in a recent study, men reported higher incidents than women, with the emergency department, psychiatry and critical care being the most common areas that abuse occurs. Nurses report more incidents than physicians and allied health workers. Bottom line is to call for help immediately if one is experiencing any threat from patients. This behavior is unacceptable in medical centers and all personnel deserve to feel safe in the workplace.

- Not planning for home discharge instructions when the patient is hospitalized. So, this issue is really directed towards those CEs who are hospitalists but can also include consultants in allied health fields asked to see the patient. Understand that the following comments are based on personal experience AND those of friends and family who have had similar experiences. Having been hospitalized twice recently, I was amazed at the lack of discharge planning on both occasions, which potentially could have impacted home care had I not been a knowledgeable physician. That circumstance should not be! As a CE and long before the hospitalist movement, I cared for inpatients a month at a time three months out of the year and taught my team to think about the patient home care needs shortly after admission, especially if there was a need for durable medical equipment (DME). Based on my recent experiences in the hospital, on one service the resident team was anxious to discharge me but were not willing or mindful to sit with me and go over home instructions. This was not a trivial issue as I had the short-term need for DME on an ongoing basis and a pain management plan. I happened to be hospitalized on a floor that did not routinely care for patients with my problem and therefore I had to sit with a caring nurse pre-discharge to go over what **I thought I needed** at home until my follow-up appointment with the physician. In fact, not all the equipment accompanied me home and my daughter had to make a last-minute visit to a medical supply house to get me the equipment I needed immediately. I really felt abandoned by the team and this hospitalization occurred at a well-known academic medical center, where the standard of care should have been higher, in my opinion. On the second hospitalization, I had questions about ongoing care in the hospital and beyond, none of which were answered prospectively by any of the team. The nurses were really caught 'in the middle' and could only relay information/questions I had to the on-call team. On that hospitalization, I received no home care instructions despite that fact that I had rib and sternal fractures suffered

in an automobile accident and testing positive for Covid-19. That hospital is affiliated with a well-known academic center in the area and again, the level of care fell
below expected standards. The physician of record, a trauma surgeon, saw me on
admission and at discharge 30 hours later and I saw the hospitalist twice. No one
even told me or discussed whether or not I had bathroom privileges and whether or
not I needed ongoing cardiac monitoring after a syncopal episode. So, not having
been appraised of these issues, I did not call for help and walked to the bathroom
myself. I attributed the limited interaction with the attending physicians and the
nurses to the fact that they were likely busy with sicker patients. I perceived that
they regarded me less ill than other patients, thereby spending less time with me.
Interestingly, when interacting with the trauma surgeon, I requested discharge as
I stated that I had been the recipient of limited nursing care and anticipated doing
well at home. His reply was hospitalization usually was 4–5 days based on my
fractures and age! I replied I was ambulating to the restroom myself and was not
being monitored cardiac-wise, so why not discharge? On discharge nothing was
stated about activity level, expectations regarding pain or when to be concerned
regarding new symptoms.

I think my experience may represent the current norm and is certainly a major
problem for elder patients who might have mentation problems and have limited
medical knowledge. Bottom line for CEs that are hospitalists: Think home
discharge planning when the patient is admitted. Discuss with the team and family
what likely will be the patient's needs at home and expectations re: pain, ambula-
tion, fever, and other issues connected with the illness. If DME or home nursing
are required, this will need to be ordered in a timely fashion if the patient is to
get this on arriving home. Finally, it is not enough to say, 'Call your doctor for
instructions regarding ongoing care', especially if discharge occurs close to a
weekend and/or a holiday. That could mean 2–3 days without meaningful interactions post-hospitalization, especially if one's doctor is not on-call, leaving the
patient feeling alone and perhaps vulnerable. Readmission in cases like this can
reflect poor planning by the CE regarding the patient's situation at home, perhaps
not taking into account the patient's limited resources. Medicare does not look
fondly on readmissions that occur within 30 days post-discharge!

- Not updating skills in interviewing. Some of us as CEs have not updated our interviewing skills, which would most likely occur at our national specialty meetings
  via workshops or through continuing education activities at our home institutions.
  It reminds me of the story by Atul Gawande in the 2011 publication of the New
  Yorker Magazine in which he speaks about the importance of coaching. He, at the
  time, was a mid-level practitioner with years of experience and upon reflection,
  decided he needed a coach to observe his performance and provide feedback to
  him. We get so into habits over time that become quite unconscious as we become
  more seasoned CEs. Coaches and others can provide us with insights into what
  we do and how we perform. I think about motivational interviewing, which didn't
  exist when I learned interviewing skills. It became a learning objective for me
  to incorporate that technique into my interviewing skills armamentarium as this
  is an important technique when one is dealing with potential behavior change

in patients. Other evidence-based information includes assessing what the main concern of the patient is and why that concerns her, Barbara Korsch's classic work on gaps in doctor-patient communication from the 60s. Interestingly that when I mention her seminal work, few faculty seem aware of her communication skills research. Bottom line is it might behoove CEs to periodically look at their interviewing skills and how they can be improved. This is more likely to happen if a peer observes you for brief periods of time and then of course, you then observe him/her/them. Having continuing professional education sessions around these techniques can be value-added to how healthcare professionals communicate. Of course, these sessions need to incorporate practice of these skills with SPs to assess what we do well and what needs to change. Being a more effective and efficient interviewer positively impacts patient care and how patients view us a professionals and human beings.

- Saying 'I don't know'. Whereas I spoke about stating this when one is teaching and is uncertain of an answer to a question, this is quite a different story when dealing with patients. One does not want to engender feelings by the patient that their doctor is not knowledgeable and/or competent. Saying that phrase in a different way can end in the same result without compromising the doctor-patient relationship. As mentioned earlier, we can be very thorough as physicians and still not be able to generate a definitive diagnosis. In those instances, we convey to the patient that he/she has perhaps not manifested enough signs or symptoms for you to arrive at a definitive diagnosis and might at that point suggest symptomatic treatment, with the patient calling in 24–48 hours to report on the progression of the disease process. With no improvement over a short time period, it is likely that testing and/or imaging studies might then be warranted. As an example, fever may be a manifestation of a lobular pneumonia that does not initially present with tachypnea, cough, rales and other chest findings (egophony, whispered pectoriloquy and decreased or tubular breath sounds). However, after 48 hours post-initial visit, the patient may indeed have some or all of those findings. Follow-up virtually or in-person is critical to resolving unknown diagnoses that initially present. So, when one has done a complete H&P and not determined the exact cause of the patient's problem, consider this status to be 'a work in progress', assuring the patient you will see this through until the problem is resolved. Better to state that despite all that you have done to make the diagnosis, it is unclear what the exact diagnosis is at this time but you have eliminated serious illnesses and are confident time will allow the disease to show itself. That is instead of saying 'I don't know'.
- Not recognizing patient's emotions upon entering the room. Often when we enter a patient's room, using the Oslerian concept of observing is key to starting the interaction. Looking at the patient's posture, facial expression and listening to her tone can all be key to how one begins the interview. It might go somewhat like this, 'Hi, Ms. Rogers (assuming you have asked the patient what she would like to be called). I am Dr. Greenberg, one of the attending physicians here, and I am happy you came in today. I noticed on entering the room that you looked sad.' After that statement, you use silence and await the patient's response. It is more often than

not that the patient will open up about her emotions and starting the interview like that will likely establish a connectedness and positive rapport with the patient. Not recognizing or acknowledging the patient's emotions might lead to lack of full disclosure on the patient's part by not providing important and sometimes confidential information necessary to make the diagnosis. The saying 'If you see something, say something' applies to medicine also. I have precepted residents who relate to me that they cannot seem to connect with the patient and almost every time it is because they have not addressed the patient's emotional state that can be obvious on entering the room. Until that is addressed, continuing with the interaction can be very difficult, especially for inexperienced trainees. Using the model activated demonstration that I previously described under Teaching prepares the trainee on what you will say to the patient in the room and how the patient will likely react. The other issue on which to be cognizant at the start of the conversation is trauma-informed care, which I discuss elsewhere.

- Assume you know what to call the patient. Looking at the name on the patient record may not be the name that the patient prefers. Once you introduce yourself, it is reasonable to ask how the patient would like to be addressed. That in itself can open up a positive and collaborative relationship from the beginning as this can be interpreted by the patient as the healthcare professional being very courteous. Some will respond using their first name, others a nickname, perhaps a few asking to be called a specific pronoun, or some a more formal name, like Ms. Somebody. Remember that the name on the medical record might not be the name the patient would like to be called. Also, in the pediatric setting, the patient's last name might well not be the primary caretaker's name so make certain you know how to address the patient.

- Silence is tolerable by most physicians. I do not believe this statement to be true, having observed many interactions in the inpatient and ambulatory settings. The average length of silence by the physician in ambulatory interactions is 18 seconds; i.e., the physician usually inquires what the reason for this visit is, the patient responds in that 18 seconds, and then the physician takes over the interview in a soliloquy, top-down fashion. This short amount of time does not allow the patient to tell her story and the focus of the interview shifts from being patient-centered to physician-centered. With the physician asking a lot of questions with binary answers (yes/no, forced choice of this versus that), the shift occurs from storytelling to responding to a set of questions, not the best way to obtain a thorough and accurate history. Physicians believe that taking over the interview, consciously or unconsciously, will save time in an environment where they are so pressed for time. In fact, not allowing the patient to tell her story is a disservice and shortcuts what the patient would like to say if being given the opportunity. Monitoring how much health professional talk versus patient talk is occurring is a way to assess if the former is doing too much talking in the interview. Practicing this skill can be reinforced by an observer using stop watches, one for the patient and one for the physician, and can help objectively assess how the talk time unfolds. Bottom line is to use more silence, especially at the beginning of the interview. If you are doing more talking than the patient, your interview can be less optimal and accurate. And by allowing the patient to tell her story, this might well provide more insights and information to the healthcare provider than by using questions requiring binary answers.

- Washing your hands outside the patient room. This, in my personal observations and as a patient, is a significant mistake. In these days of Covid-19 and other very contagious diseases (e.g., influenza, RSV, monkeypox), patients are in the position of judging physicians regarding their hygiene based on their perceptions. In fact, you might be assiduous in washing your hands in between patient visits, BUT if this is not done in the presence of the patient, it can raise questions. When I enter a room and introduce myself, at the same time observing the patient's facial expressions and body posture, I wash my hands and continue eye contact simultaneously. Whereas handshaking as you introduce yourself might not be received well by all, fist bumping can be an alternative or just a verbal greeting can be sufficient.

- The computer should not have a negative impact on patient care. It has been the norm for healthcare professionals to use the computer in patient care to preclude not being able to read one's handwriting, have better storage of medical records, allow records to 'talk' to each other (although that has been less successful in going from one medical care system to another), and reduce medical errors. The problem is that facing the computer screen and not making eye contact with the patient is a problem that can affect the relationship with the patient. This lack of eye contact might well be interpreted as not giving one's undivided attention to the patient. I suggest to trainees that they start the session, after introducing themselves, saying that 'I will be typing on the computer to document what you are saying and will not always be able to look at you face-to-face. Just know I am listening attentively even though I may not be looking at you for the whole interview.' This orientation for the patient basically addresses what will be happening and how you are very attuned to the patient's presence. It can diffuse a situation in which the patient feels negatively about this interaction. Addressing this upfront acknowledges that this model of using a computer is not ideal but is important regarding documentation and it can work even without persistent eye contact.

- Not utilizing the Korsch studies in the 1960s that addressed gaps in doctor-patient communication. I have mentioned Dr. Korsch earlier as a trailblazer regarding her studies on doctor-patient communication in pediatrics, but her results apply to all fields of medicine. Her studies involved pediatric residents at Los Angeles Children's Hospital and she found that, in most instances, residents did not ask parents what their main concerns were and why that concerned them. Those questions get to the root of what the patient/parent is worried about and need to be part of everyone's interviewing skills. To illustrate the power of these questions, we created a scenario for second year medical students in our simulation center at GWU in which a patient was presenting with shoulder pain. Of course, the students were tasked with defining the pain and using the review of systems to assess if areas other than musculoskeletal were involved. In fact, the scenario we developed was that this standardized patient worked for the postal service and was required to do a lot of lifting. He was worried that with physical therapy and treatment, he would miss a lot of work and perhaps lose his job, a significant financial strain for him. That information was NOT offered by the patient unless the student specifically asked *what* the patient's main concern was and *why* that concerned him. Basically, asking these questions uncover the main concerns of the patient versus just offering a diagnosis (e.g., rotator cuff injury) and a treatment plan, as often happens in a rushed environment. The key to this interaction was potential loss of one's livelihood and that needed to be addressed with the patient. It is easy to focus on the chief complaint and bypass what really the patient is worried about. 'Fixing' the musculoskeletal problem with physical therapy and/ or referral to a pain physician would not address the main concern of this patient, meaning the patient leaves with the same anxiety as when he came in for the visit. That is unacceptable care.

- Not offering the patient true informed consent or shared decision-making. This seems to be a pervasive problem in medicine in that not all the options for a particular diagnosis may be discussed with the patient. In fact, these options range from doing everything required for that diagnosis versus the opposite end of doing nothing. Then there might be options in-between. True shared informed decision-making implies that all possible options are outlined for the patient so that she and her family can decide on which might best for her situation, perhaps based on age, co-morbidities, living situation, finances, insurance coverage, etc. As CEs and experts, we might approach these situations with biases in terms of what **we** think is the best option, not taking into consideration the thoughts of the patient and family. Treating a particular cancer with heavy chemotherapy and/or radiation might be what the oncologist thinks is the best chance for patient survival based on collaborative cancer studies, but the patient might already be compromised health wise and not a great candidate to survive that kind of approach. I suggest that for **any** diagnosis that significantly can impact the patient's well-being, we layout all the options so there is true informed decision-making. Once that is done, I have no problems telling the patient what I would do for my own family members, understanding the patient might not choose that option. The option of doing nothing would seem anti-thetical to the caring healthcare professional, but in some instances that might be a wise choice.

- Assessing the home environment is usually considered an integral part in decision-making. As a CE working in an academic setting, my patients/families were generally from the inner city and generally had a lower socioeconomic status (SES) than people in the suburbs. Many were in inadequate housing regarding space and the environment and realizing that this can lead to some chaos in the household, it is not surprising when patients are unable to adhere to medical advice. Some of my families were living in shelters with children, depriving them of privacy and access to what we would all consider normal activities of daily living. That is not say that higher SES households do not have chaos or problems potentially interfering with their medical care and physician advice. Most of us in healthcare are from middle to upper SES and it is easy to be judgmental and/ or not considerate of environments in which people live. I remember as a resident caring for a young school-aged boy with severe rheumatic heart disease who lived with his grandmother. As a third-year resident, I decided to take him to a local professional baseball game and was invited into his home on picking him up on the day of the game. I was shocked at the meager furnishings and how he and his elderly grandmother were living. To confirm my impressions, when I was pediatric clerkship director in later years, medical students under my watch were required during their clerkship to make a home health visit with a physical therapist or nurse and were required to write a narrative about their experiences. Uniformly students reported on inadequate housing and often too many people living under one roof, affecting their daily living and healthcare. Bottom line: Ask about the home living conditions (apartment, house, numbers of people, numbers of bedrooms, presence of enough furniture, location of their housing, etc.) and support systems to assess the likelihood of adherence to medical advice. There are professionals, usually social workers and also community activists who specialize in helping to obtain better living conditions for patients and their families.

- Patients are not asked how they want information to be conveyed to them. I think we have had the experience of how patients differ in what they want from their doctor/healthcare provider in terms of how they want information provided and some of this overlaps with shared decision-making (Say & Thomson, 2003). In other words, how do they see this dyad functioning, like 'I want to know everything' or 'I trust you on decision-making so I will go along with whatever you say.' These differences can be very challenging to physicians in terms of time involvement to explain some of these issues and using the correct vernacular to explain to patients. The AMA Code of Ethics states that it is unethical to withhold information from patients, but sometimes that model can work under certain circumstances for families where an older parent is diagnosed with a life-threatening diagnosis like cancer. If the family agrees that informing the patient can be devastating emotionally and can potentially change that person's outlook on life, maybe there is room to not give full disclosure, understanding the downsides of this decision. In essence, when we meet a patient for the first visit, we should ask how they see this model playing out regarding their relationship with their doctor/health professional. My sense is based on generational differences, as older patients seem more likely to put their blind faith into how care plays out versus the younger generation seeking to be more of an equal partner. This is very patient specific, with family, spirituality/religion, health care beliefs, and age that are variables in making decisions about their wellness and disease.

- Allowing biases to interfere with patient care and decision-making. Mezirow in his theory about transformational learning, states we all have biases in everything we do (Mezirow, 1991). Those biases can be barriers in how we approach patients and their problems. As an example, if we have a bias towards a body habitus, like being obese; or a gender issue, like someone that is trans, we need to consciously think about that in the context of not letting this get in the way of our relationship with the patient or with our diagnosis and treatment plan. First impressions as Malcolm Gladwell mentions in his book *Blink* are not often accurate and shouldn't color how we think about patients until we garner more information. It's impossible and not ethical to 'hang up a shingle' that says, 'I am a surgeon but I do not accept patients who are African American or right-handed'. Certainly race, gender and lower socioeconomic status have been major areas in health care delivery and disparity, perhaps reflecting biases in some cases. Allowing these biases that we all have come to the forefront of one's consciousness as we interact with patients is very important. So, perhaps it's time we sat down and reflected on what kinds of patient characteristics make us uncomfortable and be aware of those prospectively as we deliver care that is non-biased. If ever we feel our biases are getting in the way of how we treat patients, that is the time to make the transfer of that patient's care to someone else.

- Reflection may not be a part of each patient interaction. I addressed reflection earlier in the section on teaching and it is also important in patient care. This paradigm was championed by Donald Schon and his work has been the basis for how healthcare professionals apply the concept of reflection. The 'in action' part is making certain you are in-tune with the patient as you are performing the Hx and PE. Noting any body language and/or comments by the patient may require one to state 'I noted you seem agitated and wonder if everything is ok.' This prospective awareness by the healthcare professional is key to defusing any problems noted early in the interaction. Reflection on-action is the clinical 'post-mortem' when you are basically asking yourself 'How did that interaction go?' 'Did what I say resonate with the patient and did she seem receptive to what I said?' 'Did I speak too much?' 'Would I do anything different the next time'? These all represent reflection on action. Based on my self-assessment, how does that change what I do next time in a similar situation? Again, being our own best critics on what we felt went well and what could have been done better is important in order to improve our performance over time; i.e., reflection for action. Reflective practice has made a major impact on how I have practiced medicine and taught and has also been incorporated into my non-professional life. I would suggest that making reflection a humanistic habit is a very important principle of being an excellent CE. The review article by Margaret Plack and Greenberg in Pediatrics 2005 on reflective practice really summarizes the topic succinctly.

- Trying to cover a complete review of systems (ROS) in the presence of the patient. I relate back to the early days of computers in patient care (mid-70s) when I was seen for a yearly exam at my medical school, George Washington University (GWU). To begin the interface with the healthcare system, I completed a very complete ROS on bubble paper while waiting to be seen. When I met the physician performing my Hx and PE, he addressed those areas on the bubble sheet to which I had responded affirmatively and discussed those with me in more detail (e.g., back and neck pain), omitting areas I did not consider a problem. Sometimes information like this from the patient is requested before the visit online, sometimes this can be completed in the waiting room. This information should help the healthcare provider to focus on the patient's main areas of concern, which may or may not be connected to the chief complaint. I have seen what I call the 'machine gun' ROS where the healthcare professional (often medical students) starts into a ROS that is top-down and way too fast, perhaps just trying to be 'complete' in the Hx. The patient usually answers these questions with a 'yes' or 'no' response.

Obviously a 'yes' answer deserves more detail and clarification but may be missed if the intent is just to get through this part of the Hx. The trainee is geared to 'checking off all the boxes' so that their history is deemed complete. However, there are often unanticipated positive responses to the review of systems that the healthcare professional needs to assess, determining whether they are related or unrelated to the history of the present illness in the problem-solving and decision-making process. In summary, whereas the ROS is very important in getting the complete history, devising a way to get this information in a meaningful way is paramount. I would argue this is not ideally obtained during the actual visit with the health provider but perhaps completed online or in a waiting room.

- Not having the patient undress for the exam. Both as a patient and as an observer, I have noted too many times that the patient is not undressed for the exam. I have never been certain of the reason(s) for this, but it precludes the caregiver from assessing the patient accurately. As an example, if the patient is not gowned one may not be able to observe intercostal retractions with mild respiratory distress, like with asthma or chronic obstructive pulmonary disease; or could miss an important skin lesion such as a melanoma. Having the patient wear a gown solves that problem, assuming the healthcare provider examines all areas under that gown. In addition, I have had trainees and faculty auscultate through my clothing or gown, and this is not an accurate way to perform that part of the PE. In essence, there is no reason why the patient cannot wear a gown, keeping on underwear, with the healthcare provider using a sheet as a covering, if necessary, when doing sensitive parts of the exam, like the genitalia and breast exam. In some institutions that exam may require another person in the room. With the adolescent patient, undressing in sequences, like the upper body first followed by the lower body can help allay the patient's discomfort. As caregivers, we should not be reticent to undress the patient, conveying that you will be doing a complete exam.

- Not incorporating trauma-informed care into your interaction with the patient. Using this approach can shift the focus at the start of the interaction from 'What is the reason that you came in today?' to 'What has happened to you in your past that might be of importance for me to know about?' Both questions are a reasonable way to start the interaction. So many people have had significant trauma in their past history that asking this question can open up an important conversation with the patient and guide the approach to the PE and decision-making going forward. Patients initially may often not offer sensitive information like this to healthcare givers, although they might when they feel there is trust and transparency as they decide whether or not to convey these often painful comments. Recognizing signs and symptoms of trauma-informed care in patients and family members is also important in preventing further damage that has occurred, both physical and mental health. A small but important approach is to ask the patient for permission to conduct the PE and inform the patient that you will be touching her through accepted physical diagnosis maneuvers, like palpation and use of the stethoscope. In essence, when one has lived with or been associated with an abusive spouse, parent, coach or clergy, this experience can color his/her/their behavior and emotions with the healthcare system and be responsible for why patients act/react the way they do when the PE occurs. This prior trauma can make them feel vulnerable as the CE performs the PE on them. Knowing this important information about a patient not only helps guide the CE in this exam but also helps in the counseling process going forward.

- Not addressing that you value the patient's time when you are running late. What this brings to mind is when I used to return to my hometown and accompany my late father to a subspecialist, he would say that that his treating physician always ran late and when he entered the room, would never apologize for not being on-time. Sure enough, when my Dad and I sat in the exam room for a significant period of time, his physician came in, greeted him and me (I had met him previously) and said nothing about being late as predicted. On a positive note, my previous internist (who retired too early in my humble opinion), whenever he was running late for appointments, would come into the waiting room and announce that he was dealing with a couple of emergencies by phone and apologized for being late. Bottom line—He valued my time and verbalized it in front of whomever else was in the waiting room. When you are running late because of issues with your patients, let those waiting to see you know why and that you are sorry. Patients may not know or sometimes understand why the healthcare professional is running late so explaining the reason in general terms is important. This can cause undue and unnecessary anger before the healthcare professional ever enters the room! Patients can resonate with the fact that the provider was late because of an emergency or having to spend more time with an ill patient. In fact, there could be a time that **they, the patient,** are the focus of the doctor's attention during busy office hours.

- Assessing whether or not the patient understood your diagnosis and treatment plan. This is so important as to whether or not the patient adheres to medical advice. If the patient does not understand the nuances of his health, he is less likely to follow advice. There are some simple comments that address this very issue: (1) I do not like the model of asking the patient to repeat back to you as I feel this can be demeaning. Instead, I ask how she will explain the diagnosis and treatment plan to a spouse, parent, or significant other, listening to how she interpreted my assessment and plan and correcting any misperceptions. (2) I then ask if there was anything I said about the treatment plan that the patient doesn't agree with or is unable/unwilling to do. As an example, parents have said that giving a child an antibiotic three times a day seems to be a problem as giving one dose before school or daycare and one close to bedtime is possible but a third dose mid-day seem difficult. Their schedule calls for picking up the child at 6 pm and giving the 2d dose then is an appropriate option, with last dose (third) at bedtime. The healthcare provider can make the decision of the times medication is given based on this scenario. (3) Lastly, I ask about how the patient pays for prescriptions. Whereas many inner-city families have Medicaid and older patients Medicare, that does not ensure that their insurance will cover the full cost of prescriptions, depending on a co-pay and the drug itself. In addition we prescribe many over-the counter medications, which insurance may not cover. A recent example is the cost of eye drops for my post-cataract surgery. The three prescription drops were close to $100 out of pocket, this despite my investigating the pharmacy with the best prices! And two of the drops needed renewal for ongoing care. How does the average consumer afford these prices for drugs that are necessary in the treatment? And, based on my own experiences as a patient, I found that the cost of drugs varies so widely and encourage patients with the know-how to use the internet to find the pharmacy with the most reasonable price for medications they are using. Online pharmacies in the US that I have found competitive include Cost Plus and Blink pharmacy, and these often offer drugs at much lower cost than other drug plans. Also, over-the-counter (OTC) drugs have, in my opinion, increased in price significantly over the last decade, much more than the cost of living index. OTC lubricating and antihistamine eye drops in 3 cc bottles are more than $25 each at competitive pharmacies. Of course, we as healthcare professionals cannot know the prices of all drugs but we should be alerting our patients to consider generic drugs versus name brand, and to investigate other pharmacies based on using the internet. Advocating for searching for coupons and ways to reduce medication prices is a way we can help patients financially. Even if the patient understands our diagnosis and treatment plan doesn't assure us that the she will be able to afford prescription or OTC drugs.

- Being angry when patients return for care, sometimes repeatedly, for problems we thought we had addressed accurately and successfully; and prescribed the correct treatment. Throughout the early years of my career, I remember being angry on numerous occasions when patients returned, not having adhered to my medical advice. In fact, they presented with the same complaints they had initially, these being very amenable to treatment. Perhaps in those early days, I likely did not connect appropriately with the patient as I described in one of the above points. If I established the correct diagnosis and treatment plan, the patient should be improved/improving if he had followed my advice. When patients return with the same symptoms that should have resolved with therapy, there are so many reasons why they have returned. Some of those include: (1) They couldn't fill the prescription because of costs, (2) They might not have agreed with your plan, (3) They didn't take their medication as prescribed, (4) Perhaps they have co-morbidities interfering with their treatment, (5) They have emotional issues which interfere with their focusing on the problem, (6) If they have socialization issues in their lives, perhaps they gain something positive from interacting with you and thus the reason for return visits, (7) A chaotic home environment does not allow the patient to attend to their illness or well-being, (8) They were not ready to make changes (as in motivational interviewing) in their lives at this time, (9) Their illness has persisted despite treatment. Of course, there might be other reasons but suffice it to say, instead of anger as our response and asking 'why' questions which can point fingers at the patient, we should try to determine what the reason(s) is for the return visit(s) and work from there. If, indeed the issue has to do with lack of adherence to medical advice, one should try to uncover the underlying reason(s) for this behavior. The anger we sometimes feel when patients return perhaps relates to our ego and the fact that we don't like to see negative results, reflecting on us as practitioners and suggesting failure.

- Sitting behind a desk, if indeed the exam room is set up like that. Just like in facilitating large group teaching in an auditorium where I never stand behind the lectern, I use the same principles in seeing patients. Although it may not be common in many academic settings to have desks in the examining rooms, I am suggesting never sitting behind that desk as it represents a physical barrier between you and the patient, a throwback to the hierarchy of medicine. I like to sit at right angles to the patient, not face to face, as the latter position can be an affront to the patient. Again, with the first visit, one is attempting to establish a positive first impression and a connectedness to the patient. Eliminating any physical barrier like a desk can help in that effort.
- Not using collaborative language in your discussions with the patient. I believe that using 'we' comments sends a message to the patient that the caregiver and patient are moving ahead together in a collaborative way. Again, these kinds of statements imply collaboration, trust and engagement, meaning the patient is not in this alone. 'I know you are upset, but please know I will be there for you and we are in this together.' Sometimes where this relationship can break down is during and post-hospitalization, especially if there has not been discussion between the hospitalist and the primary care physician. Hospitalists always write in discharge orders that the patient needs to contact his primary care practice. That does not always mean there has been interaction between these two caregivers during the hospitalization, perhaps suggesting that collaboration has not occurred. The patient needs to feel confident that the primary care giver and she are assuming responsibility for the wellness of the patient going forward.
- Not acknowledging that you are glad the patient came in for this visit when she did. Positive affirmation is another technique to cement the healthcare professional and patient relationship, again building trust and demonstrating that you are an advocate for the patient. It simply represents a statement one makes and acknowledges that it was a good idea for the patient to seek medical care at this time. The technique would be used mostly for sick visits and acute complaints and you are stating that seeing the patient now versus in a couple of days or a week is important to render a diagnosis and treatment that will address the problem and hopefully alleviate symptoms. In some instances, where the patient has not been seen over a significant time period, the CE can also use this statement in those cases.
- Minimizing patient complaints by affirming you have the same problem. Both as a patient and during some observations, I have noted that when the patient states 'I am having some joint pain and it seems to get better as the day wears on,' some physicians respond, 'I can relate to that as my joints are also stiff in the morning.' I say who cares what the physician has! This is not an effective way to demonstrate empathy to the patient. Perhaps a response like 'So, this sounds like it's a problem for you. Tell me the severity of your discomfort and what you have been doing for it.' Patient perceptions of what is a problem might not fit our definition but hearing the patient's story and what diagnoses are likely possibilities to explain the problem is the path to take. I am not always certain the patent cares what we as

caregivers have as diagnoses and this fact doesn't diminish the patient's concerns about a complaint she has.

- Not recognizing that the problem with which the patient presents needs more time and rescheduling for a longer visit. On some visits, especially for well children, I found that parents bring up issues that will extend the allocated amount of time for that visit, creating a backlog of patients from which one can never usually recover. Once the problem has been identified (e.g., not performing well in school, enuresis), one can certainly start down the path of getting some of the necessary information that would be pursued during an extended visit. As an example, with enuresis, a thorough history includes so many areas, including family history, sleep patterns, daytime versus night problems, etc. The PE usually does not add to the diagnosis but is important to rule out any obvious abnormalities, like hypospadias. Rushing to try to collect all the necessary information within the allotted time period can result in errors of omission and an incorrect diagnosis and treatment plan. On the other hand, allowing an extended visit to discuss the most likely diagnosis and treatment plan is preferable, both for the treating healthcare professional and patient. Informing the scheduling personnel that you need an extended visit with this patient and family is appropriate. At that point, there will be more time to establish the underlying cause for the problem and discuss these issues with the patient and/or parent. In a longer visit, one can also determine how this problem has affected the patient and family. The treatment plan is critical in this diagnosis and needs the family and child to be part of this care.
- The absence of discussion with the hospitalist regarding one of your hospitalized patients. With the electronic medical record (EMR) a commonality for specific health care systems (although there is still a problem where one EMR system doesn't communicate with others), there should be fewer communication problems and medical errors since the primary care physician (PCP) can view the patient record prospectively and before any follow-up visits by the patient. However, hospitalists may not always convey information in a timely way to the PCP and as mentioned elsewhere, home health instructions can be incomplete or not comprehended by the patient/family, short of saying that the patient needs to follow-up with his physician, the modus operandi for home-going instructions. Of course, an educated and informed patient can be proactive and make certain the PCP is aware of any problem that needs attention post-hospitalization, but that doesn't preclude the importance of communication between healthcare professionals. There needs to be a better model for hospitalists to communicate with the PCP prospectively on the hospitalized patient.
- Working in a silo and not asking input from colleagues. Whereas working in an academic setting may not be the same as in a group practice outside the institution, CEs can require 'chairside consultation' from peers when there are issues of uncertainty or even to confirm/deny a specific finding that would govern the treatment plan. That situation might happen more likely with a junior CE with less experience, but there have many times when I, as a senior physician, have asked colleagues to see my patient(s). I can remember on one occasion when I was

examining a 5-year-old, I was unable to palpate the pulses in his femoral arteries. Recognizing this would be a very unusual circumstance to not have had this previously identified and that feeling the pulse can sometimes be difficult, I asked a colleague to perform the exam without telling her what I found. She confirmed my physical finding, which is unusual at this age and suggests coarctation of the aorta. Of course, in those situations, I ask the parent's permission and explain to her that I am seeking additional 'eyes' from a colleague to see what that person thinks about a finding. One does not want to engender any doubts from the patient so a careful explanation of the goal of the additional physician visit is important. In essence, we all have had questions on occasion regarding a diagnosis or treatment plan and involving peers is often a helpful exercise. Anecdotally, I believe parents/patients welcome the fact that their physician seeks other opinions from peers.

- Not being observed by colleagues while interacting with a patient. I have mentioned Atul Gawande numerous times as a model for basically saying that he wanted to be certain that the way he was practicing met the highest standards and then some by having his former surgical chief (retired) come and observe him. One should learn from his experiences and seek out colleagues when they have protected or brief downtime to observe how we conduct patient care, receiving feedback post-observation to hear what we have done well and what we could improve. In turn, we should then do the same for the colleague observing us; i.e., observe her and repeat the process. This could be part of the culture and perhaps happen yearly for all faculty, hospitalists, generalists and subspecialists (Regan-Smith et al., 2007). This doesn't happen often enough as we sometimes assume that faulty are performing on all cylinders and not in need of fine-tuning. It would not be uncommon to hear that there is not time to do this but brief observations can be effective in generating reinforcing and corrective feedback (Greenberg, 2020). More importantly, if these observations result in affirming good practice and help to correct practices perhaps below the standard of care, that is what ideally should be the end result. The lesson here is to work smarter and not harder!

- Making certain interpreters are accurately conveying your questions and information to the patient. The need for interpreters in patient care seems to be growing as more immigrants are coming to the US, many of them as political refugees enduring hardships difficult for us to comprehend. These people come from many different cultures and speak a variety of languages. Enlisting interpreters is critical in obtaining accurate histories and providing important information about the diagnosis and treatment to the patient and family. Whereas interpreters do participate in training about medical issues, one cannot assume that any one interpreter is knowledgeable about whatever the diagnosis and treatment plan is and discussing how that interpreter is going to inform the patient is critical. Woven into this picture is how these people are living, what their support systems are and trying to make certain we recognize cultural differences. What resonates here is the wonderful book *The Spirit Catches You and You Fall Down* (Fadiman, 1997). This book involves a Hmong child and family, her American doctors, and the collision of two cultures. This Hmong family moves to the Fresno area and has a child with major neurological problems. The family's perception of the problem clashed with that of the healthcare team caring for them, to the point of involving child protective services. So, the interpreter is critical to understanding not only the issue(s) for that visit, but also how that family was living and trying to assess their health care beliefs. One of the major take-aways of the book is that it isn't just about the correct diagnosis and treatment…it's about weaving that into the culture and healthcare beliefs of the family.

- Not asking about the patient's view of spirituality, religious beliefs, and general support within their community as they negotiate life-altering diagnoses. When patients face adversity, many turn to their support systems for comfort, care and guidance. These systems can be a major source of emotional support when the patient is going through trying times. Resources can be from one's religious community, with established connections with lay leaders, church/mosque/synagogue members and/or clergy. Others have strong ties with family locally and elsewhere as a source of comfort or they also get support from close friends. Some have strong feelings about spirituality and not always from a religious point of view, but more so in awe of nature and connecting to something bigger than life as we know it. Whatever the patient's beliefs, it is imperative for the healthcare provider to determine where the patient seeks comfort and guidance and whether or not, if that involves people, to include them in the ongoing care process. This resource can be of added value as the patient struggles with her illness. These resources can be of significant assistance in coping with a diagnosis, treatment and end-of-life issues.
- Not educating patients about the ground rules of the practice. When a patient initially enters your practice, it is important to provide some kind of orientation to the practice so that expectations are clear. As a long-time academic practitioner in the inner city, I am convinced this is seldom done. Practices vary as to their logistics but there are some commonalities: (1) You will be available for most wellness or maintenance visits, with a few exceptions, like when you are on vacation and experience an illness; (2) Your availability for sick visits might be limited but one of your colleagues, including nurse practitioners and physician assistants, will always be there for you, with the medical record being accessible; (3) Defining how to reach the practice after-hours via telephone or a patient portal is very important, including some reasons why the patient should call; (4) Often-times it is social work who helps with insurance coverage and eligibility for non-private insurance, like Medicaid; (5) It should be transparent how medical coverage works on weekends and nights if one needs to be seen in-person, and that often means an emergency room visit; (6) In an academic medical center, it is imperative to define the involvement of trainees in patient care; (7) Specifying the types of visits -maintenance, sick and extended for special problems that require more time—is important for the patient to know; (8) We should also be transparent about our expectations of the patient regarding following advice, how they want information conveyed, keeping appointments, and their role as a patient; and (9) There will be times when the patient might not agree with our diagnosis and/or treatment plan and what the recourse for the patient is in those instances. In many centers

there is a patient advocate or navigator whom patients can contact when they feel they have problems with their physician or other health care provider. Whereas this list might not be comprehensive, it is a start to establishing a 'contract' with the patient, ensuring that the latter knows his rights, roles and responsibilities as your patient. This is sometimes done in the private practice world and should not differ in the academic setting.

- Not verifying what the patient has disclosed to you. This 'thinking out loud' by the healthcare provider helps to verify that person's understanding of what the patient has conveyed. 'Let me see if I understand what you said....you told me that you hurt your shoulder doing some heavy lifting and have had significant pain, mostly unrelieved by taking non-steroidal over-the-counter drugs on a regular basis. You also mentioned that you are not sleeping at night, which you are concerned that this is affecting your work. Is this correct?' Is there anything I missed?' This summation by the healthcare professional affirms what the patient has conveyed to you and if there are any discrepancies, the patient is given the opportunity to state whatever the practitioner might have misunderstood. In addition, this conveys to the patient that you are attentive and listening to what the patient is saying, promoting trust between the two parties. This should also reflect what the patient is most worried about and why she is so worried. Dealing with the patient's main concern is paramount in providing excellent care.

- Not considering written communication in addition to what you have said to the patient verbally. Invariably, patients can be overwhelmed when seeing a healthcare provider because of the information concerned with that visit. This is magnified if the diagnosis is perceived to be life-altering **by the patient**. Written information about wellness and illness-related issues can refresh the patient's memory after leaving the healthcare provider's office in the context of a more relaxed and leisure time to review the diagnosis and plan. It should be said that handouts are often found in waste baskets exiting the office if they are not accompanied by the provider highlighting and mentioning important issues on which the patient can focus. Getting the patient to relate what they have heard you say regarding the diagnosis and plan is key if we expect adherence to medical advice. Written and highlighted information can be valuable to the patient to digest at a later time. Your written information may initiate questions the patient may have that did not occur in the office visit. This written information can also be used as a guide for when the patient explains the visit to a significant other. A patient portal, now available to patients in the academic and practice settings, can also contain important information to which the patient can refer. Understanding that some of our patients are not computer literate or have access to a computer, we should be asking if they need help with the portal since this may be the best way to communicate with the practitioner.

- It's not likely social media impacts patient care. We should not underestimate the role of social media in our patients' lives, both from misconceptions of healthcare problems, unproven treatment suggestions from non-medical and medical participants (How about Dr. Oz's green coffee bean extract for weight loss or the use of Prevagen for memory loss, both products never having been studied in an independent randomized control trial?), anti-vaxers who promote untruths about the danger versus the efficacy of vaccines, trying OTC herbs/remedies that have not been studied and might react adversely with medications the patient is already taking, and promises of cancer cures that have no basis, among others. In essence, the negative impact of misinformation on social media can have long-lasting and negative effects, the prime example being the effects of measles, rubella and mumps vaccine in childhood causing autism in a bogus study published in the Lancet. In fact, the journal acknowledged this study was not valid and retracted it. However, anti-vaxers, the huge majority of whom are not health professionals, continue to refer to this study as a reason not to use vaccines. Social media seems to be the major venue in which patents receive information today about their health and some of this information is fallacious and not true. It is a good idea to check on where patients receive information about issues (like vaccines) and be ready to comment on those sources. Rather than totally negating the information they have accessed, it might be more beneficial to address why the information is not evidence-based and therefore unacceptable to the scientific community. The other issue equally as significant was the misinformation on Covid-19 virus, regarding public health prevention and vaccine protection. Preceding Covid, the Lancet article referred to above has had a ripple effect and has caused so many children to be unvaccinated, has taken decades to overturn and definitely impacted on people's views on Covid vaccine. Misinformation spreads so quickly through social media that it takes a concerted effort by public health authorities to combat these untruths. So, it is reasonable to suggest that we ask our patients where they get their information regarding their health and illness. When we know there is no evidence for a specific dietary supplement in pill form such as Turmeric, touted as an anti-inflammatory agent in health and/or disease, we need to relate to patients that there have not been any studies demonstrating its efficacy in that form. The patient can then make the decision to use or continue that supplement.

- Not considering the impact of direct-to-consumer advertising. This is a real thorn in my side issue as it gets old to hear an advertisement on TV for a drug that is being marketed to the public by a commentator speaking at 90 mph in telling what the side effects are ('If you have TB or a parasitic, please tell your doctor'), when you should call your doctor, and how great the drug is. Of course, the marketing includes wonderful 'stage effects' to draw the consumer in and convince him that he should speak to his doctor about this wonder drug. An example is Prevagen, an over-the-counter drug whose tagline is "Healthier brain, better life." This drug is formulated with apoaequorin, found in jellyfish and that actually is destroyed in one's stomach acid and never absorbed. The company states it's the "number one pharmacist-recommended drug for memory support" and in fact, is expensive since it's an out-of-pocket cost. The only studies done have been performed by the company itself, using a small sample size, and yet they advertise that the drug has been shown to be efficacious. Four years ago, the Federal Trade Commission and the New York attorney general sued the makers of Prevagen over what they asserted were false claims about improving memory and brain function. After a long delay, this suit is moving forward. This is just one example of how direct marketing to consumers can lead to inappropriate and expensive therapy, especially when the stakes medically are high. As caregivers, we need to ask patients what OTC medications/supplements they are taking as they might not even consider them drugs. When asked, patients might not even mention these OTC medications when the healthcare professional asks for what drugs the patient takes. These can have major interactions with prescription drugs. And, when they ask about ads for drugs they have seen on TV, we need to explain why that drug might/might not be appropriate for their problem, especially within the context of other available treatments.

- Not initiating hopeful discourse with the patient around diagnoses of life-altering diseases. As CEs, we deal with life-threatening diseases all too often and the way we approach the patient and family is important. Whereas we are not there to sugar-coat diagnoses that ultimately will result in death or severe morbidity, we have to look for some hope for the patient and family to hang onto, without lying or being paternalistic/maternalistic. Pancreatic cancer is a devastating diagnosis BUT some patients beat the odds, and either live longer than expected or appear, in rare instances, even cured. One of the major issues that really concerns me about end-of-life discussions is trying to predict how long the patient will live. Whereas it is important to encourage the patient to 'get their lives in order', like their finances, connecting with friends to let them know about the impending mortality, seeking guidance from an attorney, and letting family members know; in my opinion, it is inappropriate to state how many weeks or months the patient will live. Maybe stating that makes us look all-knowing, but in fact, the prediction is not always correct and unfair to the patient and family. Saying 'I don't know how long but prepare for the worst' is appropriate. That conveys to the patient that we are human and cannot predict when death will occur. The family usually focuses on a specific time we inappropriately might provide, using that date as 'This is what you told us'.

- Not recognizing healthcare disparities in patient care. So many studies have documented the disparities in healthcare for patients, many of them from minority groups and lower socioeconomic and educational status. This is perhaps part of latent institutional racism and our job as CEs delivering care to many of these patients is to be aware of these disparities. We need to spend more time educating and getting buy-in from our patients and help them in maintaining wellness and collaborate with them in addressing morbidities that are all too-common in our inner cities: cardiac disease, obesity, hypertension, chronic renal disease, poor nutrition, cardiovascular disease and others. Trying to determine how cultural beliefs can impact how patients behave is important. Using motivational interviewing as a way to make inroads around some of these chronic problems is key. Obesity is an epidemic in the US, perhaps being 'fed' by fast food access, lower socioeconomic status, lower education achievement, and lack of exercise. Until patients are ready to accept their problem and decide to do something about it, we as healthcare providers can make recommendations but these often go unheeded without the patient as a partner. Giving patients 'ugly scare' statistics on obesity for example (like increased risks of cancer, diabetes, hypertension, shortened life span), usually doesn't motivate them to change their behavior. However, showing concern about the patient's obesity and partnering with him to change his eating habits and lifestyle might go a long way to making a difference.

- Integrative medicine is not a proven entity. Some therapies considered part of integrative medicine have not all been studied in the usual randomized controlled trials we expect to see. That said, there are so many incidents where this has been the only therapy that has alleviated suffering by the patient. Patients might not always be forthcoming with volunteering that they are using some form of integrative medicine for fear that their physician will reject this, having not recommended it. Acupuncture and mind–body practices are common modes of therapy patients use, sometime without informing their physician! Yoga, biofeedback, hypnotherapy, Tai Chi, Reiki and others have attracted a large audience of patients over time, especially when traditional medicine isn't working and/or the patient doesn't want more invasive therapy. It is often used as complimentary therapy for many problems, including musculoskeletal, mental health, some inflammatory and autoimmune diseases and others. Suffice it to say this form of therapy has increased in the treatment armamentarium for many diseases, with and without the primary care physician's consent. Slowly but surely, these modes of therapy are being recognized by traditional medicine and this year Medicare has agreed to pay physicians preforming acupuncture for lower back pain. One has to assume patients have tried integrative therapies and perhaps taking OTC vitamin supplements and products promising to relieve pain and enhance immune function. Just ask the patient and you'll likely get an earful!

- Patients overreact when we convey their diagnosis. Most of life is based on previous experiences and what information to which patients have been exposed. As an example, when we assess that the patient has diabetes, the reaction from the patient may be one of shock, anger, emotional distress or silence. Another example is when we inform the patient she has a mild case of pneumonia. Of course, observing that reaction should be followed with 'You seem very upset by what I just told you'. Sometimes the patient will respond with, 'Are you certain of your diagnosis?' Of course, it would be very important to have any information available to assure the patient you are absolutely certain. You then might want to know why the person has reacted in the manner you observed. The reason could be that there are family members with the diabetes that have had amputations, chronic renal disease, visual impairment and neuropathy. With that being what the patient is most concerned about, segueing into how care will be coordinated with a physician that specializes in diabetes and a nutritionist to assist in avoiding major complications can help assuage the patient fears. In the example of pneumonia, the patient may remember people with pneumonia during Covid that had to be admitted to ICUs and were seriously ill or died. Again, explaining this diagnosis as not being serious at this stage and how it is not Covid-related can alleviate concerns. In essence, what patients deem to be serious might not be that way through practitioner' lenses.

- Some physical diagnosis skills are antiquated and not useful in patient care. I traversed medical school at a time when the Hx and PE were emphasized and that up to 85–90% of diagnoses could be made without the use of laboratory tests (Bordages, 1995). There are so many instances in my career where techniques such as percussion, whispered pectoriloquy, characterization of breath sounds, and pneumatic otoscopy have provided clear diagnoses and were value-added in my exam. In the instance where percussion may be useful, I have seen children with such enlarged spleens that using palpation may actually miss this finding if one doesn't begin the exam at the most distal part of the left abdomen (close to the iliac crest). However, percussion will yield a dull sound, indicating that the organ is enlarged. That finding can be critical in diagnosing a patient that presents with petechiae, eliminating Henoch-Schoenlein purpura and gravitating towards leukemia. In the case of suspected pneumonia, again dullness to percussion over the affected area accompanied by tubular or decreased breath sounds (depending on whether or not the bronchus is patent at that point) and whispered pectoriloquy are classic signs of pneumonia. Another PE technique that I have used consistently in my pediatric career is pneumatic otoscopy. I noted very few colleagues using this maneuver and that acute otitis media was misdiagnosed many times, resulting in unnecessary antibiotic treatment. I also found this technique to be useful in teaching trainees about the tympanic membrane (TM) and how the physiology of its movement with positive and negative pressure informs the treating caregiver. Not to be belabor the point for those of you not treating children, a TM that doesn't move with positive pressure but does come back to a neutral position with negative pressure informs us that the Eustachian tube is obstructed, most often by adenoidal tissue in young children or via allergic manifestations. The TM can be red from the patient crying but the physiology of how it moves gives us all the information we need. This is not a situation that requires antibiotics! Bottom line: Use PE techniques you were taught in medical school and beyond. I have always considered myself (humbly, I must say) as an excellent practitioner, mostly because of the training I received in medical school and the opportunity to practice as a trainee under supervision. The lost art of PE skills such as percussion and palpation in favor of more costly imaging studies drives up the cost of medicine and eliminates the wonderful feeling of success when making a diagnosis by PE alone!!! I have discussed observation previously and worry that this important part of the H&P is overlooked by the busy practitioner. Courses in art and medicine are being taught in most medical schools and observation is a key part of those courses as medical students focus on art in museums.

- What not to do if the patient doesn't agree with you. There have been times in my career when the patient didn't agree with my assessment and/or plan. In those instances, I have attempted to be persuasive about my thinking and relate that I treat my patients as I would my own family. When that approach hasn't worked in fewer than 5 times in almost 50 years of seeing patients (and I must admit it is easy to get angry about this rebuff), I have enlisted a patient advocate or representative in the hospital to speak with the patient, after I have presented the problem to that representative. The few times this has happened has been associated with the parent demanding an antibiotic or imaging study. Having a neutral person as a mediator does not always solve the problem and allow the patient/family to leave on a happy note. However, it does provide an additional contact to hear the patient's concerns and try to resolve those. What is important here is that there is an open discussion about the diagnosis and treatment plan as the patient might have some concerns that the CE needs to discuss and further explore with her. We are in a position of 'power' regarding how we assess and treat patients, BUT their partnering with us and agreeing to what we have said is a critical part of the equation. A patient advocate can be a buffer between the patient and healthcare provider and whereas the conflict might not be resolved, this model helps to assure that the patient will receive care elsewhere or via another practitioner.

- Explaining diagnoses, procedures and plans is straight-forward. I would argue, based on personal experience and that of my family and friends, that healthcare providers do NOT often speak in lay terms about some of the problems that patients experience, using way too much jargon. It is said that the average patient reads and understands at the 8th grade level. In addition, because of time factors, explaining these sometimes-complicated issues is done on a fast track, not allowing the patient to digest what has been conveyed. In addition, informed consent forms are way beyond what we are able to read, digest and more importantly understand in a reasonable period of time and to the healthcare team, are pro-forma (meaning that the patient is going to sign under the huge majority of instances regardless of what is written). That is why I have suggested a 'talk-back' in a previous bullet, making certain that the patient has a sense of what the diagnosis and plan are. If indeed there was too much jargon, there needs to be some reflection on the part of the healthcare professional to retreat and think about explaining these issues in a different way, similar to teaching a skill when the learner does not initially get it. As both a physician and patient, I also have experienced that same issue where some caregivers assume what I do and do not know. Because of the perceived hierarchy between patient and caregiver, the former may not feel entitled to question what the latter said, leaving her with questions about the diagnosis and/or treatment. Just because we are clear about the interaction going forward doesn't mean the patient is. It sometimes helps that the patient has a spouse or significant other to also hear the diagnosis and plan. Make certain you get buy-in by the patient regarding the visit.

- Not addressing that a trainee does not accurately report information about a patient or is chronically late for scheduled patient care activities. Whether this occurs on an ambulatory or inpatient rotation, the CE must address this with the trainee to determine the reason for this error of omission or commission. This error may have an impact on patient care and the overall health of the patient, reflecting on the team and healthcare facility. Setting aside time to discuss this is important to do in a timely manner. The error would have likely been pointed out prospectively and the CE would then ideally schedule a meeting with the trainee to discuss this issue in more detail. To set up this interaction, the CE might ask the trainee 'Is there a time to meet to discuss your performance on the rotation?' At this meeting, the CE might begin the discussion with 'We previously discussed and you acknowledged that you did not know all the laboratory information on our patient, and we are meeting to determine why that occurred', or 'I noted that you have been late to a number of scheduled activities, including for patient care.' Once these opening statements/questions are framed, it's important to be silent as one awaits the trainee's response. The trainee's response should verify the findings (regarding being late, not knowing lab data) and address why this occurred. In my long experience, I have never seen an issue like this denied by the trainee. Anecdotally, more often than not, the root cause of this problem is underlying issues that have affected the trainee's performance, such as illness (mental and physical), family issues (an ill sibling or parent), substance abuse, medication side effects, and other causes that would preclude expected performance. Acknowledging that this performance is below expectations is important and if there is no admitted underlying root cause, the CE should consider putting the trainee on 'probation'; i.e., give her a period of time to improve her performance on the rotation, with advice to assist her to meet expectations. This could be over three months or whatever stakeholder faculty consider to be appropriate. It is important here to emphasize that patient care is paramount; i.e., not putting anyone at risk. Reporting this behavior to the appropriate person in the chain of command (clerkship or residency training directors), alerting him/her that this trainee has been advised of the poor performance and how this needs to improve over a set time period is appropriate. Over the years, I have discovered many underlying problems with trainees that they are reticent to report, perhaps as a sign of weakness. Having an illness themselves or in a family member can have an impact on performance, and it is sad that there sometimes does not appear to be a trusting environment to divulge personal information like this. In all of my years as a CE, I have not seen similar examples in colleagues. Perhaps there is a culture where divulging personal information and how that might affect a CE's performance is not always accepted. These gaps are high stakes in medicine, especially when they impact patient care. There may be a fine line between having the required information needed for patient care or not. Recognizing this as a problem and looking for the underlying issue is important going forward.

- Eliminating Zoom visits as the 'new normal'. Covid has changed the way we have interacted with patients and it remains to be seen how this plays out in the future. Zoom and similar technology is a cloud-based app that allows the healthcare professional and patient to connect virtually without there being a visit in-person. Some patients still prefer Zoom and in many cases where a PE is not mandatory, this technology is beneficial for both parties. Mental health visits are probably the best reason to use Zoom as no PE is required. Even a neurological exam can be performed virtually with the exception of a few maneuvers, such as a reflex check, sensory exam and strength testing. Follow-up hospital visits and long-term care (e.g., CPAP use, medication check) can certainly be more efficient this way. As with many other Covid-related issues, we need more data and studies on the effectiveness of Zoom in patient care, especially if there have been gaps impacting the health and safety of patients. As studies evolve, we should pay attention to the efficacy of virtual interactions, realizing the downsides to these and examining this data going forward.

- It's not what disease the patient has, but what patient has the disease. This is an important point and one that some caregivers do not always consider when diagnosis and treatment issues are discussed. As caregivers we always have to consider each patient's circumstances when conveying diagnoses and prescribing therapy. In many instances, it's relatively easy to recognize the most likely diagnosis and treatment plan. What makes our job harder is when the patient's support system is lacking or when the environment in which he lives is an impediment to ideal care. So, as stated in previous points, making certain we know our patients and what hurdles they endure when they are not ill in addition to adding a layer of illness on top of that should color how we may treat them. I distinctly remember a case written in a respected journal decades ago about a gentleman in his 90s who was noted to have a 'spot on his lung' on a routine chest X-ray that was likely cancer. He was not a smoker and had no symptoms at that point. He related he was responsible for overseeing the care of two sisters in their late 80s and that any therapy considered would have to impact his well-being minimally. So, an interventional radiology biopsy was ruled out as was accessing the area via bronchoscopy or open biopsy. The treatment recommended going forward was focal radiation to the area, assessing its effects prospectively on the gentleman. No other therapy was considered although I could imagine that today immunotherapy might have been an option. Another recent example is an 87 year friend who has pancreatic cancer and the doctor in an academic center recommended a Whipple procedure. She is over a year post-diagnosis without surgical intervention and is doing well. Bottom line: Primum Non Nocere. First do no harm. The treatment in these cases needed to consider his age, health, responsibilities, longevity, treatment morbidity, and options that might have differed from conventional therapy in a younger person.
- Coming to premature closure on a diagnosis. This is a problem that may occur when the healthcare provider does not obtain all the necessary information from the patient, for whatever reason, or the CE's higher order cognitive thinking about the problem is faulty. Incorrect and/or premature diagnoses represent cognitive biases and can lead to delay in appropriate treatment and unnecessary testing, an emotional and financial cost to the patient. Of course, this can result in mistrust of the healthcare professional and the patient might seek care elsewhere or not adhere to medical advice, especially if there are prolonged delays in diagnosis and treatment and/or unnecessary suffering. Missing information initially can happen, but reassessing the situation when the patient is not improving is part of reflective practice. An example would be an older patient presenting with rectal bleeding, with the health care professional assuming this was the result of an external hemorrhoid versus exploring the possibility of a colon cancer that could result in a fatal outcome for the patient.
- Not doing a complete PE. This also can lead to premature closure on decision-making and result in problems for the patient. There are many examples of this, but a recent omission of a PE maneuver occurred on a baby in the well-baby nursery where the deep tendon reflexes (DTRs) were not recorded. The baby presented to the emergency department in the first few weeks of life with problems eating

and seemingly 'floppy'. There were no DTRs noted on that exam and the baby indeed was hypotonic. In essence, there were concerns about anterior horn cell disease with these presenting findings and the diagnosis of botulinum toxicity was ultimately made. Absent reflexes in the nursery should have alerted the team to this problem. It is so easy to assume certain PE findings when we examine so many patients but missing key issues like recording DTRs and a red reflex in the eye in the pediatric patient can have major ramifications for the patient. I mentioned previously about not performing a complete heart exam in trying to assess the pertinence of a murmur in pediatrics. In fact, even when we are uncertain of the diagnosis in a patient, when one has all of the pertinent information, it is so much easier to ascertain a diagnosis. Even having a peer confirm your findings is a safeguard when there is uncertainty. Doing a careful Hx and PE as if this patient were a member of your own family is a way to assure quality.

- The illogical presentation of the Hx, PE and then the lab values by trainees. This point could easily have been included under the teaching section, but I arbitrarily placed it here as this is also an important patient care issue. How trainee presentations sometimes unfold, based on my observations and experience over time, are not correct. I am speaking about presenting the history, physical exam findings and then the laboratory values. In fact, the way expert clinicians think in assessing a patient is after the Hx and PE are completed, one then synthesizes what data is apparent into a differential diagnosis, thinking about what diagnoses are most and least likely. Initially as a junior CE, this thinking and problem-solving might be characterized, as Neal Whitman, a PhD educator from Utah has stated, consciously incompetent. With time and experience, this thinking becomes unconsciously competent based on pattern recognition. **Based on the data obtained from the H&P and generating likely diagnoses,** one then decides what lab or imaging studies might be the best way to address the most probable diagnoses. For the CE overseeing patient care, it becomes easier to understand and dissect the trainee's thinking, starting with the differential diagnosis and then what labs and/ or imaging studies would be the most logical to explore those diagnoses. Jumping from the H&P to the lab tests is not the way CEs think. We always consider the most likely diagnoses, even if it is a subconscious exercise, and then determine the tests to perform.

- Not predicting what labs will show based on your diagnosis. This is another clinical skill that CEs do not always teach or adhere to themselves. As an example, if one orders a complete blood count (CBC), one can hypothesize what the results of that test will be based on the most likely diagnoses. When the patient presents with high fever and one suspects bacterial infection as the cause, it is logical to expect that white count might be high (in unusual cases low, like typhoid fever) with a shift to increased 'polys'. Regarding the hemoglobin (Hb), if the patient has pale nailbeds, it is likely that the Hb will be low. If there are petechiae on exam, one would expect low platelets although a vasculitis may be associated with a normal platelet count. We should ask trainees what they would predict regarding the lab values based on their thinking. This is an important skill for trainees to learn in order to limit unnecessary tests that do not improve care and increase costs. Sometimes we order tests because we do not really have a clear idea of the diagnosis and we go 'fishing' in order to determine the general category of the diagnosis. We are also encouraged to use panels of tests (e.g., chemistries) as this is the most cost-effective way to order some laboratory tests. Some of the tests in a panel that don't pertain to the patient's current problem(s) might reveal abnormal results and then we are confronted with do we repeat these tests or ignore them?

- Saying 'We already discussed that.' Yes, we often have to repeat ourselves, especially when it involves bad news in the patient's eyes, or when there may not be receptivity to or comprehension of the diagnosis and/or plan by the patient. If the patient hasn't heard, processed or accepted what one has said and has basically tuned us out, there will be times when we have to repeat what we thought was clear, at least in our minds, repetitively. That is why I suggested you ask the patient what she will relate to her partner, spouse, mother or significant other regarding your conversation with her and her understanding of the diagnosis and plan. I remember as a resident counseling a mother of a child with severe sickle cell anemia and osteomyelitis and on each visit, she always asked the same questions about the diagnosis and morbidity involved. My inexperience resulted in frustration versus not really determining why she was not hearing me or wanting to hear me. I probably answered in a somewhat angry tone, reiterating what I had said in previous visits and the mother likely had the same response! In retrospect, it was difficult for her to hear that her child had a life-long illness (she always asked if the sickle cell disease would 'go away') and was subject to many complications, like crises, the need for transfusions, infections, pain and growth issues. The person responsible for overseeing the development division and my training in this area at Columbus Children's Hospital (Nationwide), Steve Ruma, Ph.D. psychologist (deceased) was largely responsible for my interest in communication skills and understanding parents and patients from a developmental point of view. With experience, when patients asked the same questions that I had answered previously, I knew that there was a problem with our connectedness and I needed to revisit what they were hearing and/or understanding. Bottom line: When the patient hasn't understood our diagnosis and/or plan, we should examine how **we** transmitted that information as opposed to thinking it's the patient's problem.
- Relating that the referring doctor really did not treat the patient appropriately. This is a no–no. Whereas it may well be true that the former treating physician or healthcare provider delivered care below the standards one would expect, it is inappropriate to say that to the patient. If specifically asked, perhaps one can say, 'I treat this problem differently but everyone has his own way of doing things.' Or, 'I noted a persistent problem your former healthcare professional was treating and here is my plan to resolve this issue.' If the patient left her former practice angry or obviously not satisfied, directing blame to that practice will only inflame the situation and in the worst-case scenario, get you involved in a malpractice suit. Sometimes an incorrect diagnosis or treatment plan delays the ideal approach to the patient but other than time lost, there may be no harm that was done. If indeed a delay or incorrect diagnosis or treatment does cause harm, I believe one has to be honest with the patient and if asked, suggest that there may have been a delay

in the diagnosis and treatment. It is difficult to withhold your honest opinion of a problem missed or treated inappropriately by a former healthcare professional and may even engender some angry feelings in you. It's important to make what was wrong right and not demean a colleague. In rare instances, there could be times when there is actual malpractice with a patient you are seeing and contacting your legal team for advice is recommended as to the way forward.

- Overloading the patient with information. Sometimes we are best to provide information to patients in aliquots that they can understand and absorb versus trying to be 'complete' at one setting. There is a limit (and we don't know exactly what that limit is) to what people can hear and understand, especially if the diagnosis is perceived to be life-altering. It is known that once the diagnosis is conveyed, the patient may not be actively listening to the caregiver after that. So, providing immediately important information, like for cancer, could include that the diagnosis is undeniably correct, the treatment options are these, and what the prognosis is. Those important issues will have to be discussed again as will other nuances of the diagnosis and treatment. Having another person in the room is often helpful to make certain information that is being conveyed is being processed correctly. As mentioned earlier, asking the patient what she will tell a significant other or family member about the diagnosis and treatment plan validates what you conveyed and enables any corrections. Demonstrating that you will be partnering with the patient can have a positive impact during a difficult conversation. Lastly, having some limited written information as a handout that is succinct, bulleted, easy to read, and at a grade level that everyone will understand is critical.

- Not taking responsibility for a medical error. As former trainees it is likely we have seen errors on a regular basis during our careers, but it may not be so common to see team members taking responsibility for those errors. Since there may not have been modeling during our training on how to deal with errors, we might find ourselves confused and not certain how to respond. In today's environment, the quality improvement process and institutional legal departments are quite clear on what CEs should be doing when errors occur; i.e., report them immediately and get advice on how to counsel the patient on this issue. Modeling how to state an error was made is important for trainees to see and emulate. Importantly, learning from errors is the ultimate teaching point. Trainees should have practice opportunities with simulations (SPs) to be able to master this communication skill, a systems-based practice competency. Some errors may call for 'special compensation', such as 'I am going to give you my personal contact information because of what happened and encourage you to contact me any time'. Any deliberations with the patient would be discussed first with the legal team to determine how to best use language that would be appropriate. And of course, some errors are more 'costly' than others, resulting in unnecessary financial expenses, and/or delays in the patient getting better because the appropriate treatment and/or diagnosis were not instituted in a timely fashion. Being straightforward with a patient regarding an error demonstrates that you are human and willing to share that information with the patient, emphasizing that you have corrected the error whatever way appropriate.

- Not instructing a specialist in what you are seeking with a consultation and how you want information about a visit with your patient relayed back to you. Being specific about your referral (orally or in writing) will guide the specialist on focusing in on the problem and addressing that. Framing the referral question is critical going forward. Sometimes a telephone call or email will help define this more clearly. Although one can assume that the specialist will report all of the important findings, it is important to emphasize the team approach to that specialist and decisions about treatment and care will hopefully be decided by you and the patient once all the information is available. Whereas the consultant can provide his/her/their opinion about an issue, the ultimate decision on how to proceed with the diagnosis and treatment plan is ultimately between the CE and patient. Too often specialists provide the patient with their assessment and plan before discussing this with the CE who likely knows the patient well socially and medically. This information from a specialist can be very confusing to a patient and might not be the best approach or can even be conflicting based on all the information known to the treating caregiver. There can be many nuances that can impact treatment that only the primary CE knows and need to be considered in ultimate decisions.
- Not contacting patients in follow-up that have presented with either undiagnosed or difficult diagnoses. Making follow-up phone calls to patients who have presented with problems that concern you and them is a way to engender the collaborative approach to their care and a more empathic and trusting relationship. A day after a procedure or hospitalization, the treating professional or nurse's call about the well-being of the patient can be reassuring to her and the family as to how things are going. The same model can be employed for a patient who has an unclear diagnosis on initial exam and/or who has a serious disease. These calls need only take a few minutes and can certainly extend one's day, but the 'rewards' can be worthwhile.
- Not insuring one's handoffs are detailed. As a primary CE following a panel of patients, there are times (vacation, days off, maternity/paternity leave) when informing colleagues about your patients that need ongoing medical attention is very important if there is to be seamless continuity of care. Listing these patients with their diagnoses, anticipated potential problems, and an overview of what to expect from subsequent interactions is critical. Highlighting 'difficult' patients and families along with any nuances you feel important to convey can be very important for effective ongoing care. If you cannot be there for the patient for whatever reason(s), there often will be some expectations that care will be in-synch with what you have established in an ongoing way with the patient. Whoever assumes responsibility for a patient's care needs to make certain that first impressions are positive ones. An interaction could start with 'I know Dr. Greenberg has providing you with excellent care over the years and unfortunately he will not be available over the next 6 months as he will teaching abroad. I am very happy to be able to fill in for him during this time and encourage you to contact me when you have concerns or questions. I look forward to working with you in his absence.'

- The patient might not think of you as someone who has access to financial assistance and expertise in certain areas (e.g., school failure, housing problems, nutrition, dealing with marital issues). In fact, patients may categorize caregivers as those who treat disease and help to maintain wellness, and nothing else. Informing patients that you are there to provide services other than just diagnosing and treating disease should be established from the beginning so that when problems do occur over time, the patient feels comfortable in discussing these with the caregiver. If a parent is not aware that discussing a school problem is within the purview of a pediatrician, and that this problem may impact the child's acting out behavior, not informing the treating professional can delay diagnosis and not allow timely resolution of the problem. Another example could be that the patient has fallen on hard times and might need assistance for job counseling, food allowances and/or housing. As CEs we team with social workers and community organizations that can provide help if the patient confides in us around these difficult issues.

# References

Bordages, G. (1995). Where are the history and the physical? *Canadian Medical Association Journal, 152*, 1595–1598.
Greenberg, L. (2020). Can the recruitment of senior transitioning clinician educators enhance the number and quality of resident observations? Thinking outside the box. *Teaching and Learning in Medicine, 32*(5), 569–574. https://doi.org/10.1080/10401334.2020.1801442. Epub 2020 Aug 25. PMID: 32841577.
Mezirow, J. (1991). *Transformative dimensions of adult learning*. Jossey-Bass.
Regan-Smith, M., Hirschmann, K., & Lobst, W. (2007). Direct observation of faculty with feedback: An effective means of improving patient-centered and learner-centered teaching skills. *Teaching and Learning in Medicine, 19*, 278–286.
Say, R. E., & Thomson, R. (2003). The importance of patient preferences in treatment decisions–Challenges for doctors. *BMJ, 327*(7414), 542–545. https://doi.org/10.1136/bmj.327.7414.542

# Chapter 4
# Educational Scholarship

In this section, my intent is not to list every possible error in doing ES as that would be a herculean effort and make this section the major focus of the book. In addition, I do not possess the expertise to do that! So, my intent is to mention issues that can be significant mistakes doing ES, knowing this list is not all-complete. So, for those well-trained CEs in ES, mea culpa for not being all-knowing here. Please use additional points to generate healthy discussions about ES with junior faculty and trainees. It is also not my intent to provide details about the groundwork that was done in the late 90s and early 2000s by Boyer and Glassick in their seminal work on the definition of scholarship and how to assess that. However, I am not recommending junior CEs read their entire works (Boyer, 1990; Glassick et al., 1997). In fact, their work has also been beautifully addressed and summarized in the September 2000 issue of Academic Medicine. This information has been of major value to me in addressing ES in my career. These authors in the journal have categorized ES into areas that we can all comprehend and have importantly differentiated teaching excellence from teaching scholarship. In addition, it is very clear that the promotion and tenure committees value scholarship in the form of published studies; descriptions of curricula and models that have been studied that can be applied to other programs (the scholarship of application); non-peer-reviewed book chapters and books; and abstracts, plenary and poster peer-reviewed sessions at national and regional meetings. Whereas not all CEs see scholarship as the main focus of their careers, it is hard to be in the academic setting without doing some scholarship, even when one is on a clinical academic track. The following comments list errors that can occur around ES and suggestions on how to correct those.

- I am not certain what topic to investigate. As I stated in the published Primer in 2022, if you are a junior CE and are able to join a more mid-level or senior person in educational scholarship, that is a good way to start. However, if you are looking to find an area to investigate yourself, you have to look no further than your daily activities. So many topics have not be investigated at all, some only partially, and some might require a larger study. So many topics in medicine

L. Greenberg M. D., *Misadventures in Patient Care and Medical Education*,
SpringerBriefs in Education, https://doi.org/10.1007/978-3-031-83930-6_4

that have not been studied have been handed down from one generation to the next and assumed as fact. Other topics have been studied but there are alternative approaches that one can take that would be value-added to the literature in that area. So, I have published a lot on residents and medical students as teachers BUT had never used the flipped classroom approach to this topic, perhaps a better way to convince trainees and leadership that this approach is an efficient and effective way to teach. (Chokshi et al., 2017). Not only did this project, involving the chief residents at Children's, result in scholarship, even better is that it is an ongoing program for second year residents to expose them to knowledge and skills about teaching. The major point here is that one doesn't have to look far to find areas of ES that can be important and interesting. Being inquisitive about areas of interest in the workplace can lead one to considering studies that have perhaps not been studied or maybe only partially studied. Blending ES with one's specialty is an ideal way to approach this area.

- Not taking chances with going beyond one's comfort zone in ES. I have had many opportunities to trail blaze areas in ES, not knowing how the outcomes would evolve. The communication skills' studies I have done were all risk-taking in that I never knew if residents would participate as promised and how they would perform pre- and post-intervention. Obviously, this tentative participation can affect the methodology one chooses. Building relationships with those leaders responsible for medical student, resident and fellow education is critical to make studies like this work. Getting public and enthusiastic support from these individuals is an endorsement to which trainees will usually pay attention and increase their willingness to participate. The same could be said for my teaching-how-to-teach studies. I had conducted these initial studies as a junior CE with much naiveté in that I didn't reach out to appropriate leaders as I should have. Of course, there is always uncertainty about the outcomes if a study has no precedent. I have mentioned the book *Who Moved My Cheese?* in my book published in 2022, which addresses what the risks are for trying new and innovative programs, with no guarantees of success, versus just accepting the status quo. I loved the chance of exploring new areas and hoped that my efforts would result in enduring programs, through ES. Risk-taking is what creativity is all about and when it pays off, it can result in amazing education for participants and recognition and self-satisfaction for the CE. It also can identify evidence-based ways that specific topics can be translated into viable programs for other institutions. If you have never failed in any of your ES projects, you likely are not taking enough risks and perhaps need to reassess what ES you choose to assume. When a study does not meet the expectations of those planning it, re-looking at the data and methodology is the better part of valor, especially if one sees a significant contribution to the current literature. Thinking out-of-the-box is commendable.....just make certain the ES is focused and doable.
- Not investigating the best study design for ES. In education it is not unusual to use the single case study design in which there is no control group, and the subjects are measured at baseline and then after the intervention. This is appropriate as having a control group might not be ideal if one wants all subjects to experience

the intervention, understanding that time is valuable and that teaching, along with scholarship, is an important part of the project. There also are multi-modal approaches to scholarship in which more than one method might be value-added and reasonable. An example would be focus groups and one-on-one interviews. In this generation where many clinician educators have the knowledge about methods and evaluation, using qualitative methods is often the method of choice to study issues like communication skills, professionalism and where the N is small based on program size. If one is not expert in qualitative research, partnering with someone who has that expertise is the best way to proceed, in my opinion. If no one in the group has expertise in study design, consult with someone in the institution about this. An example of using the least ideal study design was regarding a paper I published in which we used a one-day program to teach communication skills to Critical Care fellows who deal with serious illness in children on a daily basis. All of the fellows (N = 9) participated and using standardized parents whom we trained, we saw significant change in content presented and communication skills over the one-day experience. Whereas the paper was published and has been referenced more than 100 times, the methodology of choice should have been qualitative with or without a focus group. The N was too small to present this as a quantitative study, but the data was recorded as trends rather than using p values and chi-squares. As you formulate your study and think about subjects and outcomes, this is the time to decide the best methodology considering the sample size and other variables.

- Poor articulation of the research question(s) or aims of the study. This is a trap into which we can all can fall in that we see the study write-up so many times, we sometimes overlook key wording or how this question is stated. Sometimes handing this off to a colleague to determine if the focus is clear is a great idea to confirm the clarity of the question. If the study starts out with a poorly framed research question, this indeed could be a fatal flaw and a major reason a journal rejects the paper. In addition, research questions can be too broad based on resources available and time needed to facilitate the study. Focusing in on a very clear and doable question is the key, with possibilities of follow-up studies broadening the ES. Also, making certain a complete literature review is conducted on the topic is important, especially looking at articles in how the topic was originally studied. Too often seminal articles on a topic are not included in current studies, not recognizing those that have trail blazed before us.
- Not prospectively contacting the Institutional Review Board (IRB) on a proposed study can be a problem. When in doubt, send a prospective study to the IRB for their perusal. In so many of my studies, the IRB granted an exempt or expedited status but it would be foolhardy to make assumptions about how they will assess each submission. And, it is unlikely the IRB will grant a status retrospectively if one forgets to include the IRB in the process. The review process can take a significant period of time so the sooner one sends a study, the better. It doesn't hurt to periodically ask about the status of the study in the review process just to get an approximate timeline. In addition, journals universally ask about the IRB sign off on a study. Establishing a liaison person with the IRB to discuss how

studies are likely to be categorized is ideal. I had a contact person who reviewed mostly educational studies and was most helpful in recommending an exempt or expedited review, saving significant time in getting a study approved.

- Not establishing a clear thread through the paper of the research focus, and drifting from that in the discussion. Once one establishes goals and objectives, methods and statistical design sections, all information should flow in an orderly way from those sections so that the reader can see your research process on this study in an organized approach, from stating the intent, to the methodology, the statistics, and through the discussion. The discussion should not overstate your findings, a problem I have had in some of my papers. I have also often been guilty of writing in a disorganized way and not having a logical flow to the paper once stating the goals and objectives, veering from those in the discussion. With multiple authors, these potential errors should be avoidable, as more than one person editing a paper in preparation for submission is ideal. Delegating responsibility to co-authors to re-read the paper and make edits is important. Looking at so many iterations of the paper can preclude seeing parts of the paper that need editing but one has seen too many times and passed over.

- Planning a study was beyond the resources and time available. I have always conducted short-term studies, realizing I had minimal to no funding for my early studies, that my time and that of research associates was limited based on other responsibilities, and long-term studies require a lot of resources in place. To assist in carrying out ES, I have engaged medical students and residents in many of my studies and they have been instrumental in collecting data, recruiting fellow trainees in participating in studies, and in some cases, analyzing the data. So, anytime there is data-collection, we have to work backward in time management, starting with estimating when the study will be ready for submission for publication, finishing data collection, and then crunching the data. I always defer to whomever is going to lead the study regarding timelines, letting that person set deadlines when we are to finish certain aspects of the study. Whereas some studies have gone beyond their timelines, there have been reasons for those instances and not specific to time-related issues and resources. One of the most frustrating part of conducting ES, in my opinion, is when we have been unable to adhere to set timelines. Of course, there have been many and mostly justifiable reasons for not meeting deadlines, but having data collection extend far beyond expectations is concerning, especially if collaborators are leaving for other jobs/training and no longer able to work on the project. My best advice is to get data collection in a timely fashion as other parts of the study are dependent on that. When planning a timeline, insure as much as possible that there is enough time to get everything done as determined by you and your co-authors. Recognize that unanticipated barriers will occur, and extra time needs to be factored in because of those issues.

- When a hypothesis is not supported, the authors might not be willing to try to explain what barriers might have prevented achieving this hypothesis versus an incorrect one. There have been times when the results have not been as anticipated and when that happens, we try to explain the barriers that preclude the data from being more decisive. In some cases, we have perhaps chosen the wrong hypothesis, perhaps affecting the study design and methodology. This can be a 'fatal flaw' of the study and may require a complete re-do, reframing the hypothesis. Being in this position is painful as it often means throwing out all the work to that point. Before doing that, meeting with co-authors to determine how to salvage the study is important. In addition, whereas 'negative' results are not always looked upon as a strong submission to journals, this might be a good reason to email journal editors to explain the results in an abstract and see if there is interest in receiving the study. Sometimes negative results are important to future studies and how they are designed based on how your study evolved. Then, you have to convince reviewers and journal editors of the paper's importance, most likely explaining the 'negative' results in the discussion section.

- Implying causation in a research design that is correlational or suggesting causation in qualitative research instead of developing hypotheses about causal possibilities. There are some studies that are subject to bias and nonverifiable assumptions, especially observational and qualitative studies. Having faculty with methods expertise as a co-investigator can help sort out this issue but one has to be very careful about implying causation in a study when there is no data to support this relationship. That is one of the downfalls of an observational study where there is no control group and results are based on observing behavior. Reporting what one sees is the sine qua non of observational studies but stating that results are in anyway causally related to your hypothesis can be a mistake. In the observational study by Guice et al. (2021), we observed pediatric residents asking parents for the main concern about their child's illness, and why parents were concerned, reporting out percentages of how residents performed in their interactions. We were not able to assess the root causes of how the residents communicated and future studies are the key to unraveling this concern. The study was also not able to determine what emotions parents had if residents did not assess why they were so concerned about their child. Thus, the limitations of such observational studies.

- Not making certain your confirming literature for your hypothesis and goals/ objectives going forward are laid out in the introduction of your paper. There are journal differences in how much introduction information is reasonable/ acceptable to explain your study's raison d'etre. However, the introduction provides an opportunity to review what has been previously published, how those studies might be different from this current effort, and how one will address the gaps in this study. I have found a shorter introduction works better for me regarding specifying information for the reader as to where the study is going. I then enumerate and magnify some of these differences and similarities in the discussion section. When I have worked with Ph.Ds. as collaborators, they invariably like longer introductions, a matter of style. There is no right or wrong on this difference but I suggest you check articles published in a journal to which you are submitting to determine the style of most articles. This information should help guide one regarding how to lay out the introduction of the paper.

- Not considering a theoretical construct to help explain the ultimate results of your study. Many educational journals now look for an underlying construct in papers submitted for consideration of publication. As you plan your educational study, think about exploring an underlying construct to help define your hypothesis and results. That said, I must point out that it is not clear that this approach will enhance the chances of publication. In a recent publication on retirement in academic medicine, I and my co-authors used a construct that has not specifically been applied to medicine and it was an interesting fit (Greenberg et al., 2023). I and my co-authors felt the construct enhanced the value of the results.

- Inadequate control or comparison group study. This is a major impediment when a CE works in a small program and has limited numbers of trainees to study. If one is not able to do collaborative work locally or nationally to increase the N and perhaps do a randomized controlled study (RCT), the fallback is to consider qualitative methods, single case study design as mentioned previously or a mixed methods study. I have also conducted observational studies with rigorous control of those observing, but journals are quite critical of this methodology. The fact is that I have done few RCTs studies in my career and have opted more for single case studies and less so qualitative, as that methodology was not being accepted by pediatric or other journals when I was a junior CE. The methodology and overall goals dictate how one will use statistical analysis and I have often included a 'stats person' in my studies so that I am accurate in what I report.

- Not considering the inclusion of faculty whom you think about engaging in your study but are not key collaborators in the project. On numerous occasions I and my collaborators have needed help on certain aspects of a study, often the statistical analysis and less often the methodology. In cases where we have enlisted the help of a statistician in the medical center, we have included that individual on numerous studies. In other instances, we have asked for assistance on wording of a section and/or reading part of the manuscript for clarity. If that becomes a significant time commitment, we have asked such faculty if they want to be included as an author. In addition, in studies where we have examined trainees as the focus of the study, we have asked training program directors to be co-authors to insure maximum participation of trainees.

- Not perusing educational journals to assess the kinds of articles they accept. A number of years ago there was a publication from the Northeast Group on Educational Affairs (regional group of the Group on Educational Affairs, Association of American Medical Colleges) compiled by Blanco M and Love N, consisting of an annotated bibliography of journals publishing educational scholarship. Knowing the journals available that publish such articles and their impact factor can be very helpful in selecting a journal. Some are specific to educational content, others are general journals (JAMA, Southern Medical Journal) with some educational content, and then the specialty journals that might publish occasional articles on education. First, one must have a sense of the denominator and from there look at possibilities based on the kind of article one is going to submit. Looking at table of contents in most recent issues might help in the decision-making. As an example, if the content involves residents, the Journal of Graduate Medical Education is a wonderful option, realizing that the acceptance rate is low. If your methodology and evaluation are sound, submitting to a widely read journal is ideal. The dilemma is often, in my case, do I submit to an educational journal or my specialty journals, some of which do not accept a lot of educational-oriented articles? There actually are a number of journals that focus on education but not necessarily medical education. These are journals that should be considered as perhaps second tier as places to submit only because their readership is less likely to be healthcare professionals. An example is *Faculty Development,* a journal that addresses that topic in general with minimal emphasis on medicine. However, the journal seems receptive to reviewing articles from medicine and can be a consideration if one is seeking to reach out to a more generalized audience.

- Journal editors are not interested in reviewing an abstract about a possible submission. This is variable and I have never seen a study on this. In my experience, sending an abstract to a number of possible journals in parallel is something to consider when trying to decide the best option for your paper. Journals are very competitive in seeking the submission of the best publications and some will be receptive to this outreach. The worst-case scenario is that you never hear back from the editor. Anecdotally, I once heard back from three editors, all of whom expressed interest in my paper. I submitted to one journal and another journal editor asked what the status of the paper was. I delayed writing back until I knew my paper was accepted for publication. A more recent example is that a journal, based on seeing an abstract, encouraged us to send it to one of the journal editors for a 'pre-review', meaning that evaluation of the paper at this level would determine whether or not we would formally submit to the journal. Some journals send back a pro forma answer that they cannot make suggestions without you submitting the paper; i.e., you won't have a clearer idea to submit or not based on that answer. The best answers you can receive, in my opinion, are that the article (1) does not seem suitable for the journal, thereby eliminating one of your choices. This saves so much time involved in submitting an article and then waiting for the reviews and the editor's decision. If the editor states that your paper does not seem like a good fit, one can eliminate this journal and move on, (2) The abstract sounds interesting and the editor or her designee suggest you submit the paper. The fact is that journal reviews take a significant period of time, seemingly more so during Covid, and selecting the 'right' (those most receptive based on your hearing from the editor) journal is important so as not to delay what is already a long process. BTW, receiving a positive response from an editor is encouraging but this is no guarantee of publication.
- The order of authorship and timelines for studies are areas that don't need priority discussion. When a group of CEs convene and decide to go forward with a study, it is imperative to discuss the order of authorship **from the start**. This can be a difficult conversation, depending on the 'players', especially if there is some hierarchy in those involved in the study. But in reality, it doesn't have to be a problem and one that can be discussed amiably, often led by the most senior CE. The originator of the idea for the study might not at all be the lead author, as was the case for me very frequently in my mid- and late-career stages. I often assumed the last place in the authorship, despite my having initiated almost every study.

I encourage faculty at the assistant or associate level to be first author in their quest to attain an associate or full professorship. In addition, there were often medical students and residents with whom I was involved in ES and they could be considered for first author on the paper or abstract submitted. My suggestions on order of authorship are based on (1) the work done, (2) the academic level of co-authors, (3) the number of proposed submissions for the study for abstracts and publication of the paper, and (4) the most senior author. The most senior author or the CE who assumes the lead in the study (may or may not be the initiator) should determine the author order with the input from co-authors. The lead author should be facilitating a discussion of work assignments, including data collection, statistical analysis, writing of the paper, and submission. In addition, there needs to be realistic timelines set, starting with the end in mind (submission for the publication). These should be negotiated together and carefully, understanding there needs to be some flexibility when unforeseen events occur. Someone in the group, often the most senior author, needs to be the taskmaster, making certain all uphold the agreed upon timelines. Regarding the order of authorship, this can vary from study to study. If the most senior author is a professor, that person is usually the last author, unless there is some ground-breaking study that is her idea and then she might be first. If the lead author is a junior or mid-level faculty member, that person should be lead author on the paper. Lead authorship can be important when promotion to the next academic level is considered. Tenure and promotion committees look at first authorship on ES. Medical students, residents and/or fellows might be co-authors and it is not unreasonable for one of them to take the lead on the study as has happened on many of my publications. The last variable is the number of publications anticipated from the study. This can include abstracts accepted at both specialty and educational meetings. Shuffling who is the first author on the paper and the abstracts enables more than one colleague to assume first authorship on one of the submissions and to present at national meetings.

- Funding is a deterrent to doing educational scholarship. Well, I can only relate my experience here and that may or may not be applicable in today's environment. Of course, where funds are available it makes doing educational scholarship easier. I was not able to get funding in the 80s for one of my seminal studies, teaching residents how to give bad news using standardized patients. Funding organizations replied that they wanted this study done with real patients, an unrealistic and unethical response. To have residents 'practice' with real patients was a myopic, unsophisticated and unethical look at these requests, in my opinion. I also had this happen with other projects as large funding organizations like Robert Wood Johnson and similar funding sources were not particularly interested in smaller studies in the 70s and 80s. So, looking for other small funding sources was not uncommon in my early experiences. That said, occasionally the department chair has some discretionary funds that can be used to pay a statistician or used for other expenses. I have also vied for small funds through different granting organizations at Children's (e.g., Board of Lady Visitors) and have been successful. Engaging trainees to participate does not require funding and they can add a lot to any project. In essence, the large majority of my educational scholarship (ES) has occurred without funding. I maintain that one can do short-term ES with minimal to no funds but requires some creativity using this approach. An example would be enlisting a statistician as a co-author in the study so that you don't have to pay for those services. Medical students can collect data as their part of the study and the payback is also to be a co-author. Residents often have a responsibility as part of their training to participate in research and so recruiting them for a project in which they are interested makes for a good match. Please do not allow the lack of funding to be the deterrent to doing ES.

- Not doing a thorough literature search. I have mentioned this briefly in an earlier discussion. Perhaps we have all been guilty of this but it can be embarrassing to publish an article without all the pertinent references associated with the topic. There are so many search engines that need to be accessed when doing ES, many of these we as CEs don't use frequently. I am referring to ERIC, PsycInfo, and Scopus as examples. Of course, using key words that will lead us to appropriate articles and books is important. When I have occasionally come up short on references, co-authors have added some I have not previously seen. Using the most recent articles/books and looking for references in those can also be helpful. I would also advocate for using references that described original research as those articles are often seminal in that they have stimulated ongoing studies. Many of them are quite old, often omitted, but still have significance in what we do today. As an example (without tooting my own horn), the first randomized controlled study teaching residents how to teach was conducted by yours truly and published in 1982. More recent studies often do not reference that article, and it is not part of the accessed material going forward. I find that disappointing in that the good work we do may not be recognized, assuming it adds to whatever study is being considered for publication on how residents teach. Just an example. The other caveat is developing a relationship with a medical information specialist (formerly called librarians) in the medical center and enlisting that person's help in doing reviews. I have found that to be an invaluable resource and in fact have recently published a scoping review on incivility in medical education with one of our librarians at GWU.
- Curricular innovations are not scholarship. As CEs, there are times when we innovate new curricula for trainees. If we perform our due diligence and design these curricula with rigor by including a well thought-out evaluation, there is an opportunity to publish these efforts. Many journals seek underlying theoretical constructs for the curricular design, such as Kern's 6-step approach to curricular development (Thomas et al., 2016). I remember a colleague approaching me with a curricular innovation that had been rejected by a journal, asking if I would edit the paper. After reading the paper, I suggested he insert Kern's model into the discussion, after which it was accepted for publication. It happens to be a reference that is quoted often. The bottom line is that creating a curriculum that is innovative, designed carefully and evaluated well lends itself to publication. So, when thinking about innovating a curriculum, plan ahead and encourage your co-authors to develop a rigorous evaluation and eventually publish this.

- Publishing in one venue. As mentioned earlier, there are opportunities to present your results in more than one venue. During my career, long before education was featured at my national specialty meetings, I was active in two educational groups: The American Educational Research Association, which featured a section on professionals; and The Association of American Medical Colleges, specifically the Group on Educational Affairs. The latter is divided into regions; namely, Northeast (NEGEA), Central, Southern and Western. As an aside, I strongly suggest that those CEs on North American soil check out the group in your region and attend a meeting. I have never been disappointed, having attended scores of meetings of the NEGEA and having chaired that group at one point. On many occasions, I submitted abstracts to my specialty meetings **and** to educational venues. My reasoning was that participants in these groups are very different and affords an opportunity to present study results to different audiences and receive feedback from different perspectives. Submitting abstracts to multiple meetings also allows rotation of first authorship, giving more junior authors opportunities to present before educational groups. One caveat is that it is appropriate to list an abstract once on the CV or educator portfolio even if it's accepted to more than one meeting. So, if I have presented a study at my academic specialty and the AAMC meetings, I list the presentation for both peer-reviewed meetings under one heading. Anecdotally, I remember an observational study that we had difficulty getting published initially that eventually won the outstanding graduate education presentation at the NEGEA meeting. And, a medical student was the presenter! Do you think that was not exciting for him and the team?
- Seeking 'protected time' for doing ES. When one does not have funding for a study, there is no such thing as protected time for doing ES. Even when receives a small grant to do a study, this money will not free up time for a CE. It is not possible to find a replacement for one's clinical responsibilities for one day or so a week. In fact, it is not unusual for CEs to have some limited administrative time, which often is spent catching up on the electronic medical record/patient care notations. For studies requiring data collection, I have found it helpful to enlist trainees to do this part of the study while I was performing my clinical and administrative responsibilities. However, supervising the data collection is critical as mistakes at this point can be a fatal flaw of the study. Once this part of the study is completed, getting statistical assistance, if needed, is the next step although many CEs have the knowledge and skills to crunch their own data. Again, this can happen when there are 'snippets' of time during the workday or off-hours. The same can be said for the actual writing of the paper. One of the co-authors needs to take the lead and do the first iteration of the paper-writing. Then others can offer edits, preferably sequentially, as doing this in parallel can be confusing. Bottom line is that ES is not like doing laboratory research where one needs to devote large segments of time to carry out studies that involve animals or other techniques requiring continuous physical commitment until that part is complete. ES differs significantly from this model. Again, it's important to think about small blocks of time to work on the project, more like devoting an hour or two in order to balance this with your personal life. Protected time for CEs is not findable…..don't spend

time looking for it and don't use this for an excuse for not doing ES. If one is committed to ES, one can make it happen.

- Not expanding authorship to experts outside of medicine. There are so many faculty in disciplines outside of medicine who have common educational interests with us. Some are in our own immediate academic environment, some in other universities. In fact, I have discovered faculty in business, physical therapy, physician assistant programs, laboratory medicine, linguistics, and theater/dance/motion pictures schools, among others, with whom I have collaborated. Some of those faculty were from GWU but most from other universities. Education has been the focus in each of these endeavors, with an amazing amount of learning and enjoyment accompanying the efforts. The question is how does one find people within one's own university setting or outside who are not necessarily in healthcare but have common educational interests? These collaborations have evolved in a number of ways: In a couple of studies, I noted in researching a topic there were references from faculty doing similar work in other disciplines; so, making contact to see if there was a common ground for more research was the route. In other instances, faculty attending one of my workshops often discussed the possibility of collaborative ES. These were faculty from health sciences who were involved and committed to education. In yet another instant, colleagues known to me and others have been the common contact, as was the case of the former head of the Wright State film department, Julia Reichert, who unfortunately succumbed to her cancer last year. She is the 'queen of documentaries, having won academy awards and producing such documentaries as *A Lion in the House*, on which I had the privilege of working, and *American Factory*. The former documentary followed 5 families with children/young adults with cancer from Cincinnati Children's Hospital and was a gripping portrayal of what children and families experience when cancer enters their lives. Through a mutual friend, I consulted with the group and helped organize educational modules specific to families and caregivers. These modules enabled healthcare givers to focus on specific areas, such as giving bad news, the nurse's role in a bad news scenario, and the ethical conflict of how parents of a young adult and the healthcare team struggle with stopping therapy versus continuing what is likely futile treatment. It represented an approach to focusing some of the documentary to specific categories within the documentary, attracting health care professionals who resonated with those areas.
- Giving up on a paper that you consider as being meritorious. This is one of my greatest concerns in that I have had numerous journal rejections before getting some papers published. Interestingly, the author of the Dr. Seuss books was rejected more than 30 times before finally getting published! The reasons for rejection are numerous, the worst scenario being a 'canned' answer from the editorial office of the journal stating how many submissions they receive and the small percentage of papers they accept. This would be fine **IF** they included feedback on the paper, which seldom happens, in my experience. In some of those rejections, I have specifically asked editors for feedback and almost never receive this when requested. I look at that as lack of collegiality and something every

journal should do once they reject a paper. I feel it is the journal's responsibility to enlighten the corresponding author in a few sentences regarding why the paper was rejected. How else can we learn and grow from our experiences? Sometimes we submit to a journal where the paper is not 'a good fit'. That is why I recommend sending an abstract to a number of journals in parallel to hopefully receive answers from editors to proceed with submitting the paper or not. BTW, there are no 'slam dunk' journals where you are guaranteed to get your paper published. There are, however, a couple of suggestions regarding journals that one should consider: (1) If the content is about a curricular innovation and there is some data collected to document the efficacy of the curriculum, *MedEdPORTAL* is an ideal choice for publication so that your curriculum can be replicated in other institutions. The focus in many of these articles is on the detailed process of the submission and being able to relocate the content in another academic setting. (2) If the lead author is a student, there are journals that accept submissions from medical students, especially narratives describing personal issues that impact their training. (3) A general journal which is part of the American Medical Association that accepts medical education studies and which has a large readership is *The Southern Medical Journal*. I have published in this journal a number of times and have always contacted someone at the journal to determine if my paper might be appropriate. They communicate well, in my experience, which has been helpful to me in decision-making. (4) There are journals that focus on different aspects of health and education that should also be options. Again, these journals have a rigorous review process and also consider the content of your study regarding it's fit with the journal. In the last few years, I was part of an observational study to determine if pediatric residents asked parents what their main concern was about their child's sick visit and why that concerned them. Because of the observational methodology, we had trouble getting published. Eventually, with persistence, the paper was accepted for publication and makes an important contribution about resident communication skills. There likely is a 'right' journal for your paper unless, of course, your paper has a 'fatal flaw', which if true, should be stated by reviewers.

- Not thinking about new ways to look at old subjects. Many topics seem to have been exhausted when one does a literature review, but I would argue that there are always new ways to address 'old' topics. I have mentioned teaching residents how to teach using the flipped classroom as a different spin on that topic. Other examples on which I have published are communication skills curricula for residents and aspects of empathy (in undergraduate and graduate education, career choice). Being creative in one's thinking and/or having an epiphany about a subject well-researched can lead to additional value-added studies. It is an assumption that all ES topics have been exhausted. There are always creative ways to re-look at topics of interest. As an example, there may be numerous studies that used quantitative methods to evaluate the intervention, but none that used focus groups and/or qualitative approaches. Some studies might have been conducted with a specific group of trainees, but not all trainees. There are studies that have used small numbers with interesting outcomes that need expanding upon with a follow-up study. Bottom line is to think outside of the box to expand or integrate content from one area to/ another, what Boyer and Glassick call the scholarship of application or integration. The scholarship of integration suggests making connections across scientific disciplines (e.g., business and medicine) and can result in new meaning and perspectives on topics. The scholarship of application implies connection with other disciplines to translate new knowledge into practical applications to help solve problems (e.g., applying the use of magnetic resonance imaging to use in patients).

- Not pursuing further questioning of the editor when an article has been rejected. I have questioned an editor's decision rejecting a paper on 3 occasions, two resulting in an over-ruling of those decisions (the articles were eventually published); and the other, the editors did not reply to my question. In one instance, which is one of my most referenced papers, we submitted a paper on teaching ICU fellows how to give bad news in the ICU in a one-day workshop. All eight fellows in the program participated, with the lead author being a senior fellow. Recognizing the N was small, we did not embellish our statistics but the study showed improvement in communication skills with standardized parents over the one-day workshop. The reviewers were very complimentary on the study design, but the editor rejected the paper because of the small N. I responded and told her we had full participation in the study, and with very positive reviews, and asked if she would consider sending it out to another reviewer. She agreed and long story short, the third reviewer was positive about the study and the article was accepted for publication. In retrospect, we might have considered a qualitative or mixed methods approach, but using a qualitative methodology had not had a history of being readily accepted by Pediatric journals. On a more recent occasion, we had submitted a paper on a technique integral to the ACGME competencies project. The paper originally was rejected but I agreed to make significant edits because of its importance and a resubmission after a major effort eventually resulted in acceptance. A third reply to an editor was not answered. The article I submitted was initially sent back for more edits and content revision and I immediately asked the editors if they could provide more guidance as how to revise the article, again with no response. I edited the paper as I thought appropriate only to have article rejected. Bottom line is that one does have occasional recourse when a paper is rejected to question the editor. As noted in the third example, this does not always work!!!

- When a paper is rejected, just resubmit to another journal without edits. Not infrequently early in my career, when I received a rejection on a submission to a journal, my first and obsessive instinct was to immediately find another journal to which to submit. This impulsive behavior was not smart as editors often had comments to make that were important for the re-editing of the paper. Sharing these edits with co-authors and deciding which are important to include in the paper and which are not is a critical task at this point. Some comments are dismissible and not pertinent, and others might be syntax issues that need addressing. In some instances, reviewers interpreted data incorrectly and one has to determine if that was an error on their part or not being more clear in the paper. What can drive one almost crazy is how different journal reviewers envision and critique the paper, sometimes almost 180 degrees in their comments! This can be related to the individual reviewers and/or journal style. A word of caution is that if one does not adhere to the journal format for submission, the editor might reject the paper without it ever going out to reviewers. So, make certain you have seen the 'instructions to authors' section and look at recent published articles in that journal. Focus on reviewers' comments that seem appropriate to edit areas of the paper before submitting to another journal.

- Ignoring the fact that a co-author doesn't meet deadlines or perform work assigned to her. It is a good thing that this kind of behavior does not happen often in one's career, BUT when it does, the senior author or lead author needs to speak with the involved individual and determine the underlying issue. That conversation is almost always preceded by emails and/or texts alerting everyone on the team to complete their work by a previously and mutually agreed upon deadline. Whoever takes the lead in the study represents the central repository of all the information that is happening regarding the study, whether it be data collection, statistical analyses or the actual writing of the paper. It is usually that individual or perhaps a more senior author who would approach the colleague and start a sometimes-difficult conversation. The real ultimate barrier is when a senior person on the study is the 'villain' and approaching that person might be more difficult for more junior CEs involved. In most instances, perhaps opening the conversation with 'I noticed you have had trouble keeping to deadlines on the study and wondered what is going on.' This should be followed by silence until the individual answers. In essence, you need to reinforce that this collaboration is a joint effort and that everyone needs to keep to timelines as originally agreed upon. Since this person would have been notified numerous times about keeping to the deadlines, there might be a question about his wanting to keep engaged in the study. Over my almost 50-year career, I have 'fired' three lead authors, two medical students and one pediatric resident, each of whom failed to communicate and keep me informed about their part of the study and basically were not accessible to texting or email. This after we had initially met, gone over the ground rules of how were to proceed and **they** set the timelines based on **their** schedules. Of course, I was clear that family and their medical student/resident responsibilities came first, and they were to inform me if there issues along the way that precluded keeping to a deadline. When there have been numerous communications and no responses over time and deadlines are long past, I dismissed these trainees from the studies after counseling each of them and reported this to the dean of students and the training program director, respectively. I framed this as non-professional behavior; i.e., agreeing to be an active participant in a project and not following through with communication and keeping to agreed-upon set ground rules. In each instance I expressed remorse that their behavior led to this decision and counseled them that if indeed this was not an isolated instance, they needed to change their behavior or this could have ramifications later in their careers, like negatively impacting colleagues and the worst-case scenario, patients. If this is an isolated situation, counseling should have a positive impact on them for future reference. In each instance, there were no previous incidents with any of these trainees. I have always questioned whether or not I have discovered a problem not previously recognized in each of these individuals. Of course, based on confidentiality, I would not know what happened to these individuals over time. BTW, two of three studies involving these trainees have been published and a third is in progress.

- My career is not focused on educational scholarship so I cannot get promoted based on my teaching expertise. This scenario is the case for perhaps many CEs as they are drawn to academic medicine because of their love of teaching and patient care. In their classic works in the late 1990s and early turn of the twenty-first century, Glassick and Boyer addressed the scholarship of teaching versus scholarly teaching in higher education. They also pointed out that university professors are in place to convey information and stimulate learning as one of their most important functions. They stated that separating out teaching from research or discovery was critical in terms of acknowledging what faculty do in higher education and the importance of teaching considerations in promotion and tenure committee decision. Importantly, there are the criteria that Glassick mentions in his article to assure that scholarly teaching is a distinct option for faculty. Building in reflection to this process allows the teacher to assess how things went, what needs improvement and how does one get to the point of excellence. I mentioned a story in my Primer of a mid-level faculty member who had 41-h resident core sessions devoted to her specialty topic. I asked her how she delivered this information to the residents and she responded that it was all top-down-lecturing. She stated that resident performance on patients in the inpatient unit regarding treatment had not really improved even with her providing the appropriate lecture material. Suggesting she consider changing her approach in the four sessions, I gave her a few short articles on adult learning theory and in turn, she switched her presentations to case-based interactive sessions. After doing this she noted improved performance by the residents on the inpatient unit as compared to baseline. This represents the scholarship of teaching at its best (DeSalvo et al., 2012). Of course, the fact that this resulted in two publications is evidence of the impact of the teaching innovation. Lee Shulman, a previous President of the Carnegie Foundation for the Advancement of Teaching, states that the scholarship of teaching incorporates three criteria: it needs (1) to be public, (2) to be peer reviewed, (3) to be able to be reproduced and built upon by others. One more point that I have alluded to previously. It is up to the CE to not only document teaching activities but to also specify how their teaching made a difference and perhaps led to behavior change in trainees and/or peers. I can give a very recent example of when I spent time observing residents in their Hx, PE and counseling activities. I always gave them a choice of what part of this trilogy they wanted me to observe. In fact, very few had been observed counseling patients at the conclusion of the interaction with patients and many chose counseling. Upon observing numerous residents counseling, I provided immediate feedback about this communication, invariably suggesting they make the session more interactive with the patient rather than top-down. The next time I observed the same resident, I noted that the corrective feedback I had given previously was incorporated into this interaction, demonstrating that my teaching was effective. That's the kind of experience that should be part of the educator portfolio, demonstrating one's teaching excellence. Another personal example is I have conducted a workshop on case-based teaching at numerous institutions and have discovered that some have adopted this model, again an example of how one's teaching can impact others. So, even if ES is not the major focus of one's academic career, participating in curricular development activities and/or converting teaching excellence into teaching scholarship should be considerations in advancing one's career and more importantly, making an impact on patient care or education in the center.

- Planning a workshop locally or nationally is not viewed as scholarship. Whereas having a workshop accepted to a national meeting in a peer-reviewed process is in itself not scholarship, it can evolve into that if one has clear goals and objectives, a replicable methodology and rigorous evaluation. The two examples I like to highlight are (1) the 8-step preceptor as a way to conduct case-based studies and (2) brief structured observation, a technique on how to observe trainees in an efficient and effective way. In the former example, I was intrigued with the book 'The One Minute Manager' (Johnson & Blanchard, 2003) which I felt had major ramifications for medicine. I noted that a family practice group had published a paper they called the 'one-minute preceptor', which had very little evaluation on the model they published. It was a five-step model without incorporating adult learning principles (ALPs), so I created the 8-step preceptor, which included ALPs such as learning objectives for the future. We implemented this model and studied it, resulting in a publication (Ottolini et al., 2010). As mentioned above, I have conducted this workshop using this model as an example of case-based teaching in many medical schools in N America and some faculty nationally have adopted this as part of their teaching.

The other example is a technique called brief structured observation. In the late 90s an educational group from the Indiana University School of Medicine published an abstract that presented a model that addressed the observation of trainees over a short period of time. They did not publish further on this work, and upon reading their abstract, I formulated a model that built on their work, amending some of what they presented. This represents the scholarship of application and morphed into a workshop, which uses standardized patients (medical students) to portray a young adult presenting with fever and a sore throat. A couple of volunteer residents agreed to interview the patients regarding their history of present illness with a small group of faculty observing ($N = 6$–8). I provide an introduction to the faculty, assessing why observations are so infrequent and how to orient the resident before going in the room to interview the patient, what will happen in the room, and how they will debrief exiting the room with feedback on their performance. As part of this model, I developed an encounter card displaying a checklist on the learner's performance (Ozuah et al., 2007).

The faculty are taught how to give the resident feedback in this brief observation and record their thoughts on the encounter card. This can be part of the trainee's record on a particular rotation, using this information for a summative feedback. In addition, the data on these encounter cards can be used for any ES that might be performed. I facilitated this workshop locally and nationally at many medical schools and collected feedback from participants, eventually having this published (Baumgartner et al., 2021). These are two examples of turning creative workshops and teaching methods into scholarship. Had I been keeping an educator portfolio at that time, I would have recorded the outcomes of these workshops in regard to institutions adapting them based on my intervention.

- Is it a mistake to follow a path in ES around the same general topic (e.g., teaching residents how to teach) or do I approach this more generally? In my career, I drifted to topics in ES that were most interesting to me and that I felt needed investigating, such as giving bad news and teaching residents how to teach, among others. In essence, most of my ES was focused on (1) teaching others how to teach, mindful of adult learning principles; (2) communication skills of medical students and residents; and (3) curricular innovations that have effected change. These were topics that had not been addressed often in the medical literature. Other well-published CEs have developed more vertically-oriented approaches to specific topics as part of their EP, focusing on one aspect of ES. I think you go with whichever provides you with the most meaningful feedback and enjoyment. In a vertically-oriented approach, one would be studying aspects of the same subject matter. In a horizontal or more general approach that I took, I focused on aspects of teaching and learning in a more general way that were of interest to me.

- Planning a study that involves specific individuals (e.g., residents) without communication with and/or buy-in by appropriate stakeholders. So, I will provide a positive spin on this topic to illustrate my point. In the 80s I wanted to examine residents' communication skills when a child presents to the ED dead on arrival (Greenberg et al., 1999). I realized to do this study, I needed the blessing of the residency training program director, a senior person in the department. He was not always forthcoming in giving up some control when it involved residents, so I elected to include him in the study, needing his ascent to having residents participate. This worked well and I have done that in other studies; i.e., being inclusive so that the system works well. Medicine can be very political, with faculty protecting turf. It's important to make certain that you have included all of the stakeholders in your proposed study before you proceed. It's your choice of deciding whether or not to include individuals in leadership positions to assist in the facilitation of the study. My sense has been to incorporate those individuals (e.g., a clerkship and residency program director) to help ensure the study's success. These individuals need to play a role that would help the study go forward, emphasizing the importance of the study to trainees and encouraging their participation.

- Not following journal guidelines regarding format, references and word limits. Someone as part of the team should thoroughly investigate ground rules for each journal to which you are considering submission, as they all have differences in their instructions to authors. What is fine for one journal may not apply to the others! If you do not comply with journal guidelines, they will most often either send the paper back immediately without it leaving the editor's office, or worst-case scenario, reject the paper altogether. I have written journal editors to inform them that my paper is X number of words past their accepted word limit but I don't have figures or tables. Will they accept the paper on that basis? I almost always have received a positive response. Hence, yet another reason to write the journal if you have questions. At a couple of major journals, I got to know the contact people over time as I have emailed them periodically over the years. That doesn't assure one of any increased acceptance rate, but it does give you a name as a potential conduit to the editor and the possibility of getting a preliminary response that encourages/discourages sending your paper.

- Quality improvement (QI) projects don't count as scholarship. Ever since the Institute of Medicine's treatise *To Err is Human* in 1999, there has been a flurry of activity in QI, with a mandate that departments and divisions develop projects to assure that they are striving for excellence and safety, specifically in patient care, and importantly, documenting what is being studied. Of course, we as healthcare professionals are trying to prevent errors of commission and omission. A number of journals in healthcare have evolved because of this QI system. As an historical tidbit, it is also important to know that Deming's system of profound knowledge transformed Japan post-WWII from a beaten adversary into a world leader in quality. Working with the auto industry among other businesses, suffice it to say that Deming preached the importance of decreasing variation (important when the assembly line of automobiles has to look and be the same functionally), understanding that business is a system, and realizing that the people in that system and how they function is critical. I remember that on the assembly line at the Toyota Corporation, any of the workers were empowered to pull an emergency switch IF they saw consistent problems with automobiles coming off the line. As the assembly line temporarily shuts down, a foreman would then investigate, and once the problem was identified, they fixed the problem prospectively, and avoided the recall phenomenon as has happened so often with American cars.
  So, this QI concept has been around for a long time and adapted by medicine to improve patient safety. Approaching this concept the same way you would if it were ES can lead to publications in both QI and other journals. The evaluation as an ongoing process is key in QI, assuring that gains are not just short-term and occur over time. I have encouraged rigor in developing curricula and the same model applies here so that one can not only make a difference in patient care, but also share that publicly in journals, the essence of scholarship. This effort not only improves patient care in a department and but also satisfies the requirement of monitoring that care in an academic medical center. This model to show improvement in patient care is certainly a notation one would make in an educator portfolio.
- Reviewing a paper for a journal in an area not within your expertise. Journal editors are constantly seeking reviewers as the number of submissions is growing every year, especially in education. Even in retirement, I receive 1–2 requests every month! In almost every instance that an editor sends out a review request, there is an abstract and sometimes a complete article attached. One can peruse those and decide if this is an area within your expertise to review. As an example, I do not see myself as an expert in qualitative research although some of my publications use that methodology. I know the basics of this qualitative research, but I do not feel qualified to review papers that use this method. Thus, whereas it

is flattering that editors have sought you out for your expertise, make certain you can provide a review that reflects your expertise. BTW, reviewing for journals should be included in an educator portfolio. Receiving a request to review a paper establishes that your expertise is recognized by journal editors. Finally, there are journals that are based overseas that often are online, not indexed in PubMed and desperately looking for reviewers. Many of these are for-profit journals and the charges for publications can be quite significant. I tend to avoid reviewing for these journals as they are usually unknown to me.

- Utilizing standardized patients (SPs) is a laborious way to produce ES. Having had the privilege of including SPs in many of my studies beginning in the early 80s and beyond, I am an advocate for their participation in curricular innovations to improve resident and medical student communication skills and performance. Today all medical schools have SP programs as part of the teaching and evaluating of medical students. They can be part of high-fidelity interactions based on rigorous training in their roles. In addition, I have been able to recruit standardized parents who in real life have had children with serious illnesses, recognizing they truly understand the roles they are playing. I have been able to tap into those resources and had SPs as part of such curricular innovations as giving bad news, appropriate referrals to cardiology regarding syncope in adolescents, violence screening in adolescents, and educating residents about breastfeeding. These projects were designed as curricular innovations to educate trainees about specific content areas and ultimately to be made public as ES, in essence, a dual purpose. Of course, SPs are quite used to portraying different roles with trainees and having scripts for them to learn and then practice is critical for these studies. Whereas I have not performed specific Kappa statistics to assess their inter-rater reliability, I have been rigorous in practice sessions to make certain that their responses to trainees is uniform, both in content and tone. I might also add here that standardized learners have also been an important part of my ES. These have been medical students in all instances and have portrayed patients and learners very effectively and in observation studies: (e.g., the flipped classroom in teaching residents how to teach Baumgartner et al., 2021; Chokshi et al., 2017). They not only are often willing participants but uniformly provide positive feedback about their experiences. I hope I have provided information about how value-added SPs are in our ES.
- I don't consider myself as being a good writer. Producing publishable ES mandates that you be a good writer. This characteristic is acquired by some faculty earlier in their lives based on great English and/or writing studies in high school and college. For others, it can be on-the-job training in perfecting this skill. It takes practice and input from co-authors/colleagues, not shying away from taking the lead on writing the first iteration of a study. Starting the writing of the introduction or discussion can be small steps in perfecting this skill, again having someone discussing the approach to the article and then editing your product. I have developed a writing skill that is in-synch with what journals expect but I usually defer to colleagues to check/edit my syntax and content. Not knowing the expertise of colleagues in the academic health center, it is likely there are scores of individuals within one's

own department, other departments at the medical center and university that have like interests and specific expertise to assist you in the way forward in your career. These could be content experts, like Margaret Plack, Ph.D., the physical therapist formerly at GWU who has had a major interest in reflection; a statistician who can help with methodology and data crunching; a faculty member with qualitative methodology expertise, and perhaps someone who has track record for great writing skills.

# References

Baumgartner, S., Agrawal, D., & Greenberg, L. (2021). The enhanced brief structured observation model: Efficiently assess trainee competence and provide feedback. *MedEdPORTAL, 17,* 11153. https://doi.org/10.15766/mep_2374-8265.11153. PMID: 34013022; PMCID: PMC8096882.

Boyer, E. L. (1990). *Scholarship reconsidered: Priorities of the professoriate* Carnegie foundation for the advancement of teaching. Jossey-Bass.

Chokshi, B. D., et al. (2017). A "resident-as-teacher" curriculum using a flipped classroom approach: Can a model designed for efficiency also be effective? *Academic Medicine, 92,* 511–514.

DeSalvo, D., Greenberg, L. W., et al. (2012). A learner-centered diabetes management curriculum. *Diabetes Care, 35,* 2188–2193.

Glassick, C. E., Huber, M. T., & Maeroff, G. I. (1997). *Scholarship assessed; evaluation of the professoriate.* Jossey-Bass.

Greenberg, L., Fischel, J. E., & Siegel, B. (2023). Academic clinician educators: Confronting the challenges to successful retirement. *Education for Health (Abingdon), 36*(1), 24–32. https://doi.org/10.4103/efh.efh_192_22. PMID: 38047344.

Greenberg, L.W., Ochsenschlager, D., O'Donnell, R., Mastruserio, J., Cohen, G.J. (1999). Communicating bad news: a pediatric department's evaluation of a simulated intervention. *Pediatrics,* 103(6), 1210–7. https://doi.org/10.1542/peds.103.6.1210. PMID: 10353931.

Guice, C., Schmitz, K., Aldous, A., & Greenberg, L. (2021). Observing pediatric residents' communication skills during sick visits: Do they determine caregivers' main concern and their reasons for concern, and are caregivers satisfied? *American Medical Student Research Journal, 7*(1).

Johnson, S., & Blanchard, K. (2003). *The one minute manager.* Harper Collins.

Ottolini, M., Mirza, N., et al. (2010). Student perceptions of effectiveness of the eight step preceptor (ESP) model in the ambulatory setting. *Teaching and Learning in Medicine, 22,* 97–101.

Ozuah, P. O., Reznik, M., & Greenberg, L. (2007) Improving medical student feedback with a clinical encounter card. *Ambulatory Pediatrics, 7*(6), 449–452. https://doi.org/10.1016/j.ambp.2007.07.008. PMID: 17996839

Thomas, P. A., Kern, D. E., Hughes, M. T., & Chen, B. Y. (2016). *Curriculum development for medical education: A six-step approach* (3rd ed.). Johns Hopkins University Press.

# Chapter 5
# Promotion and Tenure

This process in academic medical centers is a way for CEs to be recognized by their peers for their expertise in any of the foundations of the mission statement. It also can be linked to salary increases, recognizing one's excellence and rewarding that individual appropriately. Tenure is not a likely track for most CEs because of their significant patient care responsibilities, and therefore most CEs will be on some kind of clinical track. Based on one's personal mission statement upon entering academic medicine (and realizing this can change over time), this will usually identify the focus of a CE within the center. It is the CE's responsibility in documenting excellence in that area (or areas) so that those on the Tenure and Promotion committee can assess the worthiness of promotion for that individual. Keeping an educator's portfolio and having a mentor to advise you in this important area of being an academician is crucial.

- Not **negotiating** an academic appointment, salary and fringe benefits when one is approved for a job at an academic medical center. For many of us, this becomes a moot issue if this is our first academic endeavor. It is likely the offer will be at the instructor or assistant professor level. It may be, however, that there is flexibility in funds available for an online degree in medical education or for advancement in one's career in teaching through workshops offered by the AAMC or other like organizations. In essence, when the center has offered a position, one does have some leverage in negotiating salary and possible benefits to enhance one's career. I have always maintained that it doesn't hurt to ask…and to stick to what one believes is the right path. The recruitment process can be quite costly, and it is likely there is some flexibility in what the center is willing to offer, but you have to ask! However, if one is simultaneously being recruited by another academic center for a new position, one can use that leverage to negotiate academic position, salary and fringe benefits before taking a position.
- Submitting a CV for promotion purposes unaccompanied by an educator portfolio (EP). I have reviewed many curricula vitae (CVs) of CE faculty up for promotion and too many have been unaccompanied by an EP. If the major focus of a CE is not

ES, then there must be documentation regarding what the CE has accomplished, and in my opinion, that is rarely reflected in a CV. I have responded to the point person sending the CV to please enclose additional information that would be found in an EP. It seems not all academic health centers require an EP, which seems to be a disadvantage for those faculty not focusing on ES. The purpose of an EP is to not only list educational scholarship and patient care activities that characterize how effective the faculty member is, but it should also provide information about how that faculty member has promoted behavior change and influenced trainees and colleagues through their efforts. As mentioned previously, relying on traditional evaluation forms with Likert responses are inferior to narrative forms that provide more details about that CE's performance in order to make an informed decision about promotion. I am not suggesting that a CV is not important, just that it alone does not characterize the effectiveness of the faculty member. Listing the number of lectures one presents does not address faculty effectiveness and their impact on trainees. The same can be said of the number of mentees one has engaged. Commenting in a narrative how one has advanced the careers of mentees is how an EP compliments the CV.

- Being considered for promotion prematurely. There have been times when a CE requests being considered for promotion, which perhaps may be premature based on available documentation. This decision on pursuing promotion should involve the faculty member's mentor and/or the person in charge of faculty affairs within the free-standing department (e.g., children's hospital) or the medical school. Knowing the standards for promotion is very important as is assessing one's documented activities as compared to those standards. Whereas the promotion and tenure committee can provide constructive feedback on one's performance over time, it is sometimes deflating to hear that your promotion has been denied, meaning a 'rejection' by your peers. So, I recommend that a CE discuss promotion issues with a mentor or head of faculty affairs as these individuals are always willing and able to provide sound advice around this issue. Again, I have been asked to review CVs for people considered for promotion (that I do not know) and often see limited documentation of activities, especially around patient care and administrative areas. ES is easier to document and becomes part of the 'bean counting' for promotion and tenure committees; i.e., abstracts, oral presentations and published papers that are peer-reviewed and accepted for publication and then book chapters and/or books themselves. Areas outside of ES need more specific documentation as to how the particular issue (e.g., teaching) impacts trainees/peers.

- Not reading and understanding the rules in the faculty handbook on tenure and promotion (P&T). Tenure is not an issue for the huge majority of CEs promotion and each institution/department has a set of ground rules on criteria for promotion to each academic level. It is incumbent for each CE to read and understand those rules before proceeding in the promotion process. This is a mistake that CEs can make, especially if they have a mentor who is not involved in the process and who also might not know these criteria. Reflecting on the criteria and determining where one stands in the process is first and foremost. This exercise can alert CEs as to what gaps they need to plug in their CV regarding these criteria and what the promotion and tenure committee will be looking for.

- Vague guidelines in the faculty handbook on promotion and tenure. This can be a major problem, especially when CEs' expectations regarding promotion do not happen, even occasionally leading to lawsuits if this area is not specific. Faculty also have to be responsible for making certain their documentation for their performance is objective and clear to the committee. I originally was denied promotion to professor in the 80s with a strong CV (almost 50 peer-reviewed publications, many abstracts and presentations at national meetings, book chapters, and national recognition in medical education) because I was informed that committee members were not familiar with the educational journals in which I published. These were all mainstream journals in education and certainly known to educators in the field. In retrospect, I might have predicted this as none of the P&T committee had published in education nor would they have read any of these journals. It just didn't happen that way in those times. I would hope that those making decisions about promotion today are more aware of educational journals in which CEs publish.

- Letters of recommendation supporting your promotion. Although obtaining strong letters of recommendation need not have to be emphasized, I would suggest that these letters should not reiterate what is in one's CV but highlight and summarize one's strengths for the promotion committee. As an example, if teaching is the major focus of the candidate, then providing both anecdotal and objective evidence of teaching excellence should be the major part of the supporting letter, outlining how that teaching has contributed to the department/institution/medical school or even nationally. The candidate should provide those who are writing supporting letters important information about his/her/their career path and evidence of why they should be promoted. Having an educator portfolio accompanying one's CV should enhance the available information that will be used to make the decision and I consider that a must (It is never too late to start an EP, documenting what you do educationally, administratively, scholarly activities, patient care-wise and mentoring going forward). Of course, if the candidate has transformed teaching excellence into teaching scholarship, that is even stronger evidence pertaining to that candidate's readiness for promotion. I would also suggest that when asking for a supporting letter, it is important to determine if that person can write a really strong letter, which would be very important for promotion. There might be times when the person asked to write the supporting letter is not able to comment about the candidate in the superlative. The candidate should be frank and ask if the faculty person is able to write a strong letter. On occasion, I have related to the requesting CE, with some difficulty, that I am unable to write the strongest letter for promotion based on the information presented to me. If asked, I can outline what issues fall short in going to the next academic level. The decision to ultimately have me write a letter falls to the faculty member.

- Not informing those who wrote letters for promotion on your behalf of the decision. So many times I have written supporting letters for faculty (some of whom I have never met!) for promotion and have not heard of the decision by the promotion and tenure committee or the candidate of the decision. Do I really have to state that it is a common courtesy when colleagues write letters for you to inform those faculty of the decision? When I was not promoted to professor the first time, I let my supporters know and they were incredulous, wanting to know how they could help the next time I was up for promotion. They provided the most supportive letters the next time I applied.....and I was promoted! Promotions are not automatic and informing those who wrote letters if you were not promoted can be guides to what additional information they should include in a subsequent letter.

- Being first author on papers is not important. In fact, tenure and promotion committees often look at first authorship when assessing a CE's request for promotion consideration at the associate and professor levels. When one ascends the academic ladder, CEs need to take the lead in ES and curricular initiatives; and assuming first authorship on any final products submitted for publication or inclusion in a school or program curriculum **is** important. Reviewing CVs where the candidate has not had many first authorships on publications makes me question that person's leadership capacity, creativeness, organizational skills (perhaps not able to definitively delegate ordership of authors) and input into those studies. First authorship usually connotes that the candidate has assumed responsibility for the study and facilitated carrying it out. Once one reaches the professor level, unless the study is groundbreaking, there is no need for CEs to be first author. I have previously addressed how CEs collaborating in a study negotiate authorship, recognizing there might be numerous opportunities for first authorship on platform presentations, posters, and the actual paper.

# Chapter 6
# Administration

Very few faculty in the past have received any formal education during their medical school and residency training about the administrative functions that are required to meet the mission statement of the institution, department or medical school. That seems to be changing with time as faculty are recognizing the importance of addressing what knowledge, skills and attitudes are integral to carrying out these non-patient responsibilities. Some faculty actually pursue MBAs as a way to further their expertise and ability to attain higher administrative positions within the medical school, department or private industry. Whereas this body of knowledge and skills seems to become more important as we ascend the academic ladder, in fact many times junior CEs are appointed residency training program director or clerkship director, often with little attention to the knowledge and skills required of these jobs. I have noted over time that many of these areas in leadership skills are offered as workshops at national meetings, giving participants opportunities to learn and practice skills. Some of these involve running a meeting, conducting focus groups, brainstorming ideas, overseeing employees working under us, creating a budget, being knowledgeable about strategic planning, implementing projects, balancing responsibilities between faculty and professional leadership, problem-solving an important issue, and much more. Bland et al have written a seminal book over 30 years ago on how faculty can be successful in their careers, with a section on the administrative domain (along with other previously addressed issues (Bland et al., 1990). This textbook is relevant even today. It is hard to ascend the academic ladder without assuming some administrative activities in the center.

- Not developing a personal mission statement. In my opinion, this is a very important part of defining yourself as a professional and CE. I suggest that one does this in 30 words or less, which is a most difficult task. It takes introspection to do this and makes one focus on one's priorities as a CE. That said, it also allows the CE to examine new opportunities by looking at one's mission statement to see if this new opportunity fits where one is at professionally. Another caveat is that the mission statement is subject to change over time, especially as the CE matures in

L. Greenberg M. D., *Misadventures in Patient Care and Medical Education*,
SpringerBriefs in Education, https://doi.org/10.1007/978-3-031-83930-6_6

her career. Maya Angelou's 'mission statement', which she framed as her goals in life, is a wonderful example. "My mission in life is not to merely survive, but to thrive; and to do so with passion, some compassion, some humor, and some style."—Maya Angelou. My own initial mission statement was that whatever I did in medical education, I wanted to make a difference. That goal was before I knew anything about mission statements and defined me as to my commitment and passion.

- Not having the right skills for an added responsibility. So, as we go from junior CEs to mid-level and beyond, it is likely we will be asked to assume new responsibilities within our division, department and/or medical school. What often comes with these new responsibilities are leadership and management tasks, many for which we have received little or no training. As an example, overseeing faculty within a division requires an understanding of management issues, conflict resolution, facilitating a division meeting, counseling (and more counseling, of faculty), and juggling a budget within the mission statement of the institution, division or department. These skills are generally not taught in medical school and residency training, and faculty gravitate toward advanced online MBA degrees and/ or national specialty meetings are featuring some of these topics as a continuing professional education experience. Perhaps a most difficult area are the skills in counseling fellow faculty who have life and developmental crises (divorce, pregnancy, death in the family, retirement, parting from a long-time relationship as examples) and need to express their concerns about how this has affected or perhaps will affect their career. This can take significant time and not having the necessary skills to listen and know when to possibly refer an individual to someone with more expertise can be a problem for the involved faculty member and leader. In addition, these kinds of problems can sometimes result in personnel shortages, requiring others in the division/department to pick up any slack based on this scenario. Other examples would include leading a meeting as a newly appointed chair of a committee or task force. Again, there is a science to how to lead an effective meeting and sitting through one in which the chair of a committee does not seem prepared or to have done some necessary outside work prior to the meeting can be deadly, and more importantly, a waste of faculty time. There is a major difference between running a meeting and facilitating a meeting. In the former instance, it is creating an agenda to which **you** adhere, creating the goals and objectives, talking most of the time, and a top-down approach. On the other hand, facilitating a meeting generally has participants coming prepared, like having read material ahead of time; being inclusive; promoting active participation, and getting your 'covert' agenda through, making the committee members seemingly making that happen and not you. As an example, I chaired the pediatric clerkship committee and having read some key evidence-based information, decided it was time to have the clerkship scheduled educational sessions transform from lectures into case-based interactions with the medical students. I presented 'my case' before the committee and let their discussion dictate how we should vote, with the committee overwhelmingly agreeing to change the format. I hope you can see the parallel in how this approach is the same I have advocated regarding how we teach. Importantly, when one is selected to assume a new position and is aware that this new responsibility will require a different skill set, negotiating with leadership that you will want to attend courses to achieve these skills is important upon accepting the position. I understand when junior CEs are offered positions like clerkship or residency director, they might feel unempowered to respond to senior CEs that they need training in administrative skills and that needs to be part of the offer. I maintain that if leadership has agreed you are right for the job, negotiating for further training should not be a barrier.

- Not negotiating some discretionary educational funds to use for journals, meetings and professional enhancement. If you are THE candidate for the position (assuming there were others that applied), it is clear that the institution wants you as a faculty member. If you are making education your focus, maybe specifically teaching, it is reasonable to convey that to the interviewers and that the purpose of these funds will be to enhance your knowledge and skills in education. I cannot imagine the reply being that that can't be part of the contract. I can assume that the only sticking point might be the amount they will allot you. So, do your homework, and find out the yearly costs of journals (e.g., Academic Medicine, Teaching and Learning in Medicine) and annual meetings that feature medical education (e.g., regional Group on Educational Affairs meetings, specialty meetings). Also, make certain you are clear about having your department pay the cost of any meeting in which you will be presenting a poster, workshop or abstract. These issues need to be negotiated upfront and not after you have been at an institution for a while. To my dismay, I have recently heard that some institutions are not paying faculty expenses when they have had peer-reviewed abstracts, posters and platform presentations accepted at national meetings. To avoid confrontations retrospectively, one should negotiate these in initial contract discussions. Don't underestimate your negotiating power!

- Not staying abreast of current policies and policy changes. Things are changing so fast in medical education and patient care that keeping up with policy changes and how they affect current practice in day-to-day academic life is critical. Although 'old hat' now, the competencies and milestones in residency training created a major impact in how faculty assess resident education and performance. Theoretically, this model is a better mousetrap in assuring the public we are turning out physicians that we are certain have attained entrustable professional activities and are competent. However, there are many more studies necessary to document that this model is indeed effective. The competency project of the ACGME has been a work in progress and a monumental effort to get faculty buy-in. In addition, residents and students are stakeholders in this change in the way we evaluate trainees and I have found them often uninformed about the competencies and milestones. As an anecdotal example, when I have asked a trainee what competency/milestone is involved in her interaction with the patient and perhaps within the context of the teaching point, they uniformly have given me the 'deer-in-headlights' look. I maintain that the competencies and milestones are part of their training and they need to be informed. More recent concerning problems are states' laws in the US that have been enacted on gender and abortion issues, affecting training and care. How medical schools and departments address these laws/policies is another example of moral distress, meaning how do we serve our patients' needs outside of government regulations? Policy changes should lead to faculty development efforts and other forms of educating faculty around specific topics. Failing to communicate changes effectively to faculty can lead to mistakes in patient care and education. Also, these policies can affect career choices of medical students and faculty need to be prepared to discuss these issues as they impact our profession.

- Not negotiating salary when you accept your position. I have addressed this point in my *Primer (2022)*. Those in HR and/or your division that want to hire you usually have a range of salary they are willing to give you in the hiring process. Of course, you may not be privy to those range in salary numbers, just know they exist. There are two factors here that should encourage you to negotiate a higher salary: (1) You are offered the position so the institution values you, has chosen you over other candidates and wants you to commit, (2) This should bolden you and not let you underestimate your self-worth. When a salary is offered, I would suggest a moment of silence and reflection, eventually responding with 'Thank you for that very nice offer and I appreciate the institution's/division's support. However, I was hoping to receive more in salary when I considered the position.' I don't see this as big risk-taking as they might reply that this is the highest amount they can commit. Then you have to decide to opt-in or out. Asking for a few days to reflect on the offer is also not unreasonable and something you might want to discuss with a significant other, attorney or a friend in the business world. With likely room to increase the initial offer, HR may increase the amount if the institution wants you. On the other hand, if that is the 'drop dead' salary they have committed to this position, be ready to accept it if they reject your request for an increase in starting salary. This initial offer should also be addressing academic funds for furthering one's career as I mentioned in the *Primer.*

- Not having a game plan for implementing change. When I began my career as a CE focusing on education, I realized that effecting change around educational issues was a major hurdle. It was not enough for me to be passionate about what I did….I needed to develop strategies to make change happen. A major strategy was making certain colleagues were familiar with educational literature that I made available. I coined the term 'covert infiltration' as my modus operandi to effect change, through daily conversations, workshops, committee meetings, modeling, ES and mentoring. I believe that I did effect change based on feedback I received over time and the fact that my CE colleagues assumed more responsibility for evidence-based teaching and learning. I also recognize that there are barriers within any institution over which one does not have control that makes effecting change difficult. Again, thinking about strategies on how to get others 'on-board' with perspective changes is critical. Also recognizing that change takes time and does not happen overnight is important to recognize as academicians often look for immediate results. The most memorable change that happened on 'my watch' was being part of the transformation of the Department of Obstetrics and Gynecology at GWU to teaching, starting with a residents-as-teachers program and progressing to the full-time faculty (Greenberg et al., 2016). This involvement with residents initially and then having faculty engaged was a strategy that worked and more importantly, has resulted in lasting change. Educational principles can be foreign to faculty in that they have not been exposed to terminology and theories that promote more effective and fun learning. Introducing these principles and their applications can be so illuminating as a 'new' way of teaching, attracting attention to an area not previously addressed.

- Accepting your salary without questioning as you progress up the academic ladder. There are times when you have accomplished some innovative work, not only enhancing the division and department but being recognized nationally for your efforts. This occurred when I started the Office of Medical Education at Children's in 1978, a full-service office across the continuum of medical education. The Office, through mostly my efforts and those of my continuing professional education director, became widely known in educational circles and 12 years into my work, I asked the Chair of the department whether or not my salary at that time was 'fair'. Essentially, he told me to 'benchmark my work'; i.e., determine what other like offices/CEs were doing and how they were remunerated. Knowing the field in Pediatrics, I told him it wasn't likely I would discover someone elsewhere doing the same things I was, and I was correct. Two younger colleagues doing less than I were being paid up to $50,000 more a year. This benchmarking resulted in an increase in salary for me and would never have happened had I not challenged the Chair. Reflecting on your accomplishments on your career path and questioning your remuneration is a model that certainly occurs in the business community. We are often rewarded on our performance through promotion and less so financially, unless we raise the issue.
- A detailed job description is not provided to you orally or in writing, including items you might have requested, like money for continuing professional education in a specific area or travel for professional reasons. Once you sign on the dotted line, a contract is a contract and if all the details about which you spoke, negotiated and requested are not there, one has lost an opportunity. Promises made orally don't always work or are acknowledged as administrations and leadership can change very quickly. Details about what you have discussed and were seemingly approved need to be explicitly present in the contract. Unfortunately for CEs, contracts contain so much legalese that if one needs assistance from an attorney that can help with understanding the wording, it's often worth the price. Sometimes a friend who practices law can peruse the contract and provide some advice on how to proceed. Bottom line is to make certain all the issues for which you have negotiated are part of the contract before you sign. Unfortunately, this is all about business and no place for oral agreements or promises. Lastly, your specific job description in writing is so important as there can be areas of misunderstanding that are communicated orally but don't appear as you assumed in the contract. One of the first responsibilities to which I was delegated as Vice Chair for Education was to create a strategic plan for faculty development. I did my due diligence based on my knowledge in the field and experience and after a significant effort, presented this to the department chair. He did not agree with my approach and

had other ideas on how this was to work, creating a divisive relationship from the beginning.

- Being asked to meet with someone in a leadership position and not knowing the agenda. I have mentioned this in the Primer, but this cannot be stated enough times. When invited to a meeting by someone in a leadership position, ask what the agenda will be ahead of time so there are no surprises. If the agenda is not clear to you, ask clarifying and/or probing questions so there are no 'grey' areas before your meeting. One doesn't want to attend a meeting where you are asked to do something that is not of interest to you or to assume a position that you are not seeking. When attending a meeting where there is no agenda or it is not clear, leaders from a position of power may 'arm twist' to have you do something you do not want to do. Also, forcing one to make a decision at that point without time to reflect and determine how this will impact one's current activities is to be avoided, understanding leadership called you to a meeting because they are invested in you. Of course, referring to your personal mission statement to see if whatever is offered fits your best interests is also very important. I was offered the Chief Medical Officer position after temporarily assuming that role, with a major salary increase. I declined after considering my mission statement and spousal input. So, best advice based on personal experience is to make certain what an agenda is BEFORE attending a meeting with upper leadership and do not feel forced to accept a position or proposition until you have taken time to reflect on that offer.

- Avoid delegating as this gives you less control. One of the keys to my success as a CE was that I was able to hire administrative assistants (AA) who were quite capable and willing to accept responsibilities that more senior people or faculty do. A classic example was collating medical student narrative summaries for their clerkship grades and presenting them to me for my edits. Invariably, this task in the past was always assumed by the clerkship director. Before I delegated this responsibility to my AA, I taught her what I was expecting and she accepted this without hesitation. In essence, I didn't ask the AA to editorialize but to only collate what the narrative would look like along with the final grade. This is what we sent to the dean of student's office at the end of a rotation. The only edits I ever seemed to make was when the evaluation was not balanced and included only corrective comments but no reinforcing ones. I had the AA send that narrative back to the faculty person writing it and suggested that comments on things well-done be included to present the evaluation in a balanced way. This was one example of something I delegated that freed me up to do other important tasks. In fact, I knew of no other clerkship director in North America that used this model. Another example is that I oversaw was continuing professional education (CPE) and delegated that responsibility to a person in the office, a Ph.D. with expertise in medical education. I allowed this individual to propose educational activities and shared my thoughts with him/her prospectively. Both individuals who held the position were very competent, making the delegation of this part of the office much easier. Again, establishing relationships, setting ground rules upfront, and making certain we were on the same path regarding goals and objectives were all important in making this delegation work well. It was nice to know that I had a smoothly running CPE office while I was able to focus on other issues. The same model occurred for overseeing all educational activities in the hospital, with an AA that accepted responsibility for this task.

- Develop a working and collegial relationship with administrative assistants that work with you. Whereas I was their boss and had the responsibility of evaluating their performance, I have always had a wonderful relationship with my AAs and very little turnover during my career. In my 22 years as founder and director of the Office of Medical Education at Children's, I had three AAs over that time period. I remember one asking me why she worked so much harder than other AAs around her. I told her that in my search for excellence, it required lots of effort on everyone's part, working as a team. Once she heard my explanation, she was obviously satisfied with that and remained with me until my retirement from Children's. The keys to successful relationships with AAs are the following, very similar to the relationship of the teacher and learner: (1) trust, (2) clear goals and objectives, (3) delineated roles, responsibilities and expectations, (4) perceived diminished hierarchy, (5) team effort, (6) honest and timely feedback, (7) ability to effectively communicate, and (8) a safe environment.
- Not addressing gaps in performance in AAs working under you. When I started the Office of Medical Education at Children's in DC, I had a number of people whom I supervised, including the head of CME and those AAs that staffed graduate and undergraduate medical education. Periodic evaluations of those personnel were part of my responsibilities and I had to provide objective and helpful summative feedback to them. On rare occasion I had to relate constructive comments to one of them regarding gaps in her performance that needed addressing. In one instance I had been telling my AA for graduate education about the importance of timely filing of reports, on which she always procrastinated. I finally had to tell her that this had reached an impasse requiring me to inform Human Resources (HR) about this issue. With counseling, this AA improved her performance and this issue was resolved. Had this not been the case, I had documented our meetings and discussions by email and had involved HR along the way. Whereas I, of course, didn't pay her salary, she and others in the Office were under my supervision and I was the one evaluating them.
- As CEs we don't always have a lot of say about how money is spent in our divisions, especially when it involves education. In academic medical centers our divisions are not expected to be profitable revenue centers, rather to meet budget expectations. Getting involved in budget planning at this level enables one to potentially influence how money is spent each year as opposed to leaving this function to others. Being able to interpret and prepare financial reports is a skill that also carries over into grant funding. Top-down approaches to the budget are commonplace where senior leadership sets the budget for the yearly cycle. Obviously, this has to be in-synch with the institutional budget. As CEs we may not have a lot of leverage to impact budgets and areas that we feel need more funding or any funding at all. That is not to say we shouldn't offer our input on the budget cycle, especially around issues involving education. Being somewhat

knowledgeable about the budget for your division is something you can do and benchmarking how other divisions in the region budget for similar services can be helpful.

- Not paying attention to finances. In addition to your salary, you have other benefits through your department and/or medical school that you need to be aware of. Some of these may include life insurance, which may not be enough to protect your family should something unexpected happen to you. The same can be said of disability insurance and know that payments to you are not tax-free if you are disabled and have not paid the premiums (as opposed to the institution paying that). Thus, one might consider seeking advice about taking out separate policies to cover your family needs should you become disabled or die. This is not my area of expertise, but I think that there is a direct correlation with age and the amount of the premiums; i.e., the older one is, the higher the premiums for disability and life insurance can be. In terms of the profit-sharing that is part of the fringe benefit package at most N. American institutions, the department/medical school usually contributes to your retirement plan by matching what you contribute up to a certain limit. This is 'free' money and one should think about making a maximum contribution if you are able. How that money is invested can be an issue so getting financial advice regarding your investments is an option. Some CEs have invested poorly and upon retirement, do not have the funds required to enable them to have a worry-free life. Also, one has to consider financial obligations such as carrying for aging parents and helping our children, the sandwich generation. Bottom line is to pay attention prospectively to this important area and not assume anything.
- Not having leadership and management skills can be a deterrent to accepting a leadership position in the division, department or medical school. There are so many issues facing CEs in the academic setting, many of them in administrative areas as our careers advance. Faculty face ambiguity, stress, conflict and overload in regard to their responsibilities of fulfilling the mission statement. Those in positions of power need to be self-aware of their leadership styles (Myers-Briggs Type Indicator) and how those potentially impact others. Without these skills, CEs will find their jobs more difficult as they go up the academic ladder. I have seen accomplished faculty attain leadership positions without these skills and that has resulted in problems in governing.
- Not being aware of the relationship between the department, medical school and university. There are so many models out there as to the inter-relationship of these stakeholders, and it is important for leaders to understand their complexity as none exists in isolation. There can be conflicting demands for resources and limitations placed on each of these entities, making understanding how they function in relationship to one another and the negotiating power each has is important. There are practice plans totally separate from the university and medical school, with the latter contracting with the practice plan for teaching. As an aside, I remember a former business-oriented GWU President talking about eliminating the medical school so as to 'improve the bottom line' at the university and what implications that would have for the hospital, the Medical Faculty Associates group (practice plan) and affiliated departments, like the free-standing Children's Hospital. There

did not seem to be any consideration of the stakeholders that would be involved in this decision, not the least of whom would be patients in the inner city and region affected by this top-down decision. Again, recognizing that decisions can have a ripple effect and impact those stakeholders downstream is a reality.

- Uninformed about how to create a strategic plan. Having the knowledge and skills to create a strategic plan is important for more seasoned CEs as these are blueprints for divisions, departments and medical schools in projecting where they want to be in the next 5–10 years in regard to the mission statements of each entity. This requires thinking out of the box, being knowledgeable about health-care and educational systems and being creative in terms of how to affect change. An example was when the current chair of Ob-Gyn at GWU wanted to change what was perceived as a hostile learning environment in the department and Jim Blatt (a valued internist colleague at GWU) and I negotiated facilitating a series of resident-as teachers workshops as the starting point. We then wanted to see if there would be a ripple effect that impacted faculty and resulted in sessions on teaching and learning for them. These workshops were well-received by the residents and the effort evolved into a publication (Gaba et al., 2007). Interestingly, the faculty in the department also became curious about this effort and the curriculum segued into one for the faculty through grand rounds and practice opportunities. In essence, this informal strategic plan resulted in significant change in the department and national reputation as one invested in education. The department used this change to market how it recruited for the residency program, emphasizing the focus on education.
- Paperwork is annoying and not something to spend quality time on. Based on my interactions with those in academia and private practice, paperwork can consume us and takes a significant period of our time, not likely reimbursable. (Paperwork today is mainly in the form of the electronic medical record). That being said, that does not change the importance of careful documentation regarding our interaction with patients and our administrative work. Documenting what we have done and writing about that process is key to good patient care, especially when there are ongoing medical problems and specialty colleagues involved with our patients from time-to-time. This careful documentation helps to assure a complete and safe handoff. These principles also apply to our administrative responsibilities, like our managerial role with people in our workplace. This would include evaluations over time and helping these employees to succeed with timely and pertinent feedback.
- Excelling in each cornerstone of the institutional mission statement. I believe the days of the 'triple threat' are over, when the CE was able to excel in patient care, teaching, ES and advocacy. When one formulates a personal mission statement, which should reflect and identify the focus of one's professional being, this will likely include an area of focus such as ES or patient care. As mentioned earlier, this can change over time as one ascends the academic ladder. CEs are best served to focus on an area of excellence and build their educator portfolio based on that. Being a jack-of-all-trades in today's environment is much harder than in the past as opposed to having expertise in a specific area. Of course, one plan is to devote a certain percentage of time to each of the areas of the mission statement, with

one area being the major focus. Teaching and patient care often consume the huge majority of any CE's time.

- Lacking facilitative skills in leading small or large groups. As we assume leadership responsibilities, we are often asked to lead groups of peers or others in problem-solving important areas via committees or task forces. This can include brainstorming, paired weighting, action learning, problem-based learning, and other evidence-based processes to facilitate small group decision-making and learning. These tasks have specific applicability to different situations and the leader needs to have an armamentarium to use as needed. Some of these skills are defined and detailed in books and others can be learned from peers at workshops locally and nationally. Being aware of nuances that make small groups work, like speaking to group members individually before any meeting to sell an idea, are important skills that facilitate accomplishing an agenda. It is critical to have group members feel valued in the group and to have a vested interest in seeing the group succeed. This well can become 'community' for group members, feeling connectedness to each other.

- Not responsive to texts, emails and/or phone calls. This topic really doesn't fit in any of the categories I have listed but has always been an area of annoyance to me. Whereas expectations shouldn't be unrealistic regarding how soon colleagues should respond, I would offer that any response at all is collegial versus no response, which has happened far too often in my career. Perhaps it might be that those who feel less 'attached' to us don't always feel obligated to respond, but I have often sent repeated texts or emails and not heard back from faculty with whom I have a relationship and some only in passing. I find this behavior of ignoring correspondence as unprofessional and in fact, if this occurred with trainees where they didn't answer, we would call them out on this behavior sooner than later. I would guess we seldom do that with peers if at all. We are all busy, and in many instances, very overcommitted regarding the responsibilities we have. That as a given, we should still be professional and respond to communications from peers in a 'timely' fashion. Besides being unprofessional, lack of response usually demonstrates no interest in the topic **or you** as the sender! And yes, communication can get lost in cyberspace, but not repeated communications.

- Not planning for retirement. As a senior CE, retirement is inevitable, sometimes based on health issues, age, other interests and/or disenchantment with one's career. While planning for eventual retirement, the CE needs to connect with the department chair to inform her of one's retirement plan in the near future. If the CE wants to stay connected to the medical center in some way post full-time work, either in the department or the medical school, he should negotiate in advance for part-time opportunities or options to continue in a voluntary capacity. For CEs, opportunities in teaching, mentoring, patient care (on a limited basis) and advocacy could be possibilities. For those with no interest in continuing connections with the academic center, looking at volunteer opportunities outside of medicine is advisable.

- Finding a way to say 'no' when asked by a more senior person to assume an administrative responsibility. As an example, if a more senior member of the department offers you what seems to be an exciting administrative opportunity, reflecting on your mission statement and deciding whether or not this request 'fits' is important. On reflection, stating that the offer sounds very interesting BUT not within your mission statement up until now is a reasonable and thoughtful response.

# References

Bland, C. J., Schmitz, C. C., et al. (1990). *Successful faculty in academic medicine: Essential skills and how to acquire them.* Springer Publishing Company.

Gaba, N. D., Blatt, B., Macri, C. J., & Greenberg, L. (2007). Improving teaching skills in obstetrics and gynecology residents: Evaluation of a residents-as-teachers program. *American Journal of Obstetrics and Gynecology, 196*(1), 87.e1–7. https://doi.org/10.1016/j.ajog.2006.08.037. PMID: 17240248.

Greenberg, L., Blatt B, Keller J And Gaba N (2016). Can a residents as teachers program impact a department's educational transformation? *Journal of Faculty Development, 30*, 41–45.

# Chapter 7
# Mentorship

This section is shorter than the others but that is not to devalue its importance. Mentors are such an important part of academic life as they help less experienced faculty to grow professionally, offering advice and more importantly confirming what CEs need to hear about their plans/goals. Mentors can be tapped locally or nationally and usually are in the same field as the mentee, although two of my main mentors were Ph.Ds in education. I have also engaged giants in the education field along the way in my career who offered counseling on specific issues and thus never had a long-time relationship as is typical in a mentoring relationship. In fact, I **never** had any of the leaders I met in medical education ever turn me down when I approached them, saying a lot about the learning climate in those early years (70s and 80s). Mentors offer specific knowledge, skills and experiences so the mentee has to be clear what she wants from the mentor. A mentor can help with mission statements, long- and short-term goals, conflict management issues that occur, monitoring progress, balancing professional and personal life and helping that CE to be self-sufficient with time. A major reason for a mentor is to have someone monitor one's professionally activity and assure that the mentee is on a path to excellence in a particular area; e.g., patient care. This striving for excellence is a way to be promoted, feeling self-worth and being recognized by peers in doing that. I distinctly remember a valued colleague who excels in providing the most complex care to children with multiple disabilities once state that she didn't really care about the promotion process. I countered her by saying that it is a major way that peers show that they value what we do. I know that is not what we are trying to achieve as our end result and that self-satisfaction knowing you have contributed to the patient and family is paramount. However, in an academic setting, the promotion process is inherent to rewarding one who excels in a specific area(s) of the mission and should reinforce what we inherently already know as great work. Mentorship helps us along that path. As a disclaimer, the reader should recognize that mentoring is different than coaching. The latter involves a relationship between two individuals with the faculty member being coached already having expertise and wanting to focus on an area on which to improve. The examples

L. Greenberg M. D., *Misadventures in Patient Care and Medical Education*,
SpringerBriefs in Education, https://doi.org/10.1007/978-3-031-83930-6_7

of coaching I have used previously include Atul Gawande's search for excellence through the eyes of his former department head and the model of observing each other in teaching and patient care that I mentioned.

- Mentoring comes easy like teaching and is not an area in which you need training. Mentoring skills are not innate. I know that some CEs have personalities that enable them to connect to learners in a meaningful way. However, I see mentoring skills in a parallel fashion to teaching in that there is a body of knowledge and skills that have been extensively published in peer-reviewed articles and books that need to be incorporated into the mentoring process. In my national meetings in Pediatrics, I have seen a significant increase in workshops offering these skills and knowledge with opportunities to practice in simulated situations that can enable CEs to be better mentors. I am concerned that faculty who mean well volunteer to become mentors and have no such training. Each department/division should establish as one of the prerequisites for being a mentor is to have a specific level of training and there should be opportunities to learn these fundamentals in workshops with hands-on experiences. Approaching mentoring should be viewed similarly to teaching: (1) identifying a body of knowledge that has evolved from ES on the topic; (2) determining how one would apply that knowledge in the clinical setting; (3) seeking workshops that focus on the process, with practice opportunities to learn these skills; and (4) thinking about using your mentoring experience to transform into ES. In essence, it is not enough to have content expertise in a specific area to be a competent mentor. One needs the skills and knowledge of mentoring that are delineated in the literature.
- You only need one mentor. Perhaps this is true for some CEs, but I would counter that in many instances, one mentor does not fit all. Over my career, I had a number of mentors, each of whom offered me something a little different. One of my first mentors, the head of education and the pediatric clerkship at Columbus Children's Hospital (now Nationwide Children's Hospital), was a wonderful mentor, stayed in touch with me when I left my residency, and told me there was always a place for me at the hospital had I decided to return. A second mentor was a Ph.D. who served as the first head of CME at Children's in DC and was instrumental in my learning important principles about ES that I never learned in medical school or residency; i.e., research design and methodology, statistics, and other nuances of research. She was instrumental in our being funded for our study on teaching residents how to teach, the first randomized controlled trial reported in the literature. We wrote many papers together and facilitated numerous workshops nationally. She really was a major factor in getting me on the path of my career in medical education. A third mentor was a visiting professor at GWU on a number of occasions and introduced me, through his workshops, to being an effective lecturer. He also was a Ph.D. in education and was responsible for my visiting the Center for Educational Development (now the Department of Medical Education, the University of Illinois) on a number of occasions to attain building blocks in medical education. It was there that I read numerous books on teaching and learning and curriculum design, and discussed some of these issues with

wonderful and receptive faculty. The last mentor I wanted to recognize was a fellow pediatrician and educator who believed in me and really pushed me beyond what I thought were my limits. I had been nominated for the chair of the Northeast Group on Educational Affairs (part of the Group on Educational Affairs, the Association of American Medical Colleges), which consists of the medical schools from Canada down to the Washington area. I lost that election and this mentor **told** me forcefully that I was running for the chair again. I replied that losing the election was a message and that didn't sound like a great idea. He would not take 'no' for an answer and I was fortunate to have won the second time around, being the first CE elected to that position. There are mentors that can assist the CE on the following: (1) gender modeling, (2) ES, (3) source of knowledge, (4) networking locally and nationally, (5) providing feedback, (6) trusted relationship, (7) good listener, (8) problem-solver professionally and personally, (9) key to career success as a CE, (10) sharing rich experiences, and (11) academic promotion (Choi et al., 2019). Choose those that best fit your academic and personal needs.

- Not acknowledging what your mentors have done for you. Unfortunately, we sometimes take for granted what mentors do for us as CEs and don't thank them enough. Perhaps that occurs because of the sometimes short relationship that the dyad has had, focusing on a specific problem that has been brought to closure. Also, not seeing or interacting with the mentor on a regular basis as we navigate our busy workdays could be another reason, some of them being from other institutions. As we segue from one CE level to the next (especially as we become more senior), there might be less need for a mentor and out-of-sight, out-of-mind. Whatever the reason(s), make it a point to thank those who mentor you as a demonstration of appreciation for how they have impacted your life as a CE. This can be communicated whatever way you wish....I vote for a more personal touch like by phone or if able, in-person, or maybe at a national meeting over lunch. I reflect on this point as I recall numerous times when someone I mentored briefly and some more intensively thanking me for my efforts and how I impacted their teaching, ES and/or career. More often than not this happens serendipitously through another context, but this may be reality as people tend to forget what is not currently impacting them. Much of my career successes I can attribute to receiving advice/counsel from a mentor. Don't forget their investment in you as a CE and reach out to them to thank them for their assistance in molding your career.

- Building a trusting relationship. This is key to mentoring. Developing rapport and empathy as part of this trust-building are important components. Listening to the mentee and understanding her goals and needs also helps building this relationship. Upon reflection, I realized that all of my mentors had many of the characteristics that are important in developing trust. This made it easier for me to speak about my gaps in knowledge and skills as I knew they would not be judgmental. My experience is that upon entering this new relationship, the dyad may really not know a lot about each other, personally or professionally. Relating about one's pertinent experiences in life is a great way to break the ice and get to know one another. In addition, there will be potential topics addressed there are sensitive and confidential and both parties need to respect this as part of the trusting relationship. Again, there are so many commonalities in the mentoring process in how we relate to patients and how we engage our learners. Trust is of the essence in getting to really know and understand our mentees.

- Not making time to observe the mentee. I am not certain how many mentors observe their mentees, but I would consider this an integral, although perhaps atypical, part of this relationship. Of course, this is not logistically possible when our mentors are not local. This can be so valuable as I have mentioned in the sections on patient care and teaching as part of a CE's growth. This can be collegial and not top-down once there is trust established between the two. These sessions, perhaps occurring twice a year, can be so value-added for the CE and experiences that can be logged in an educator portfolio; i.e., I was observed doing a history by my mentor and was offered the following constructive and reaffirming feedback, whatever that might be. With time always being a limiting factor, using the model of brief structured observation described earlier can be an efficient and effective way to observe. The mentor can glean important information observing the mentee that can be related back to her to further that person's growth around patient care. This model crosses over into coaching although it might lack the depth and breadth of what coaching is intended to be.

- The mentee does not always provide both reinforcing and constructive feedback to the mentor. Well, this has happened so many times in my career where I have given up valuable time providing advice and counsel to a mentee, including writing a powerful and thoughtful letter of recommendation for a mentee, and never hear back on the impact of my mentoring. So, am I not making the ground rules clear? Does the CE for whom you write the recommendation not see your involvement as investment in the process? Is this simply an error of omission? Is this rudeness and not showing appreciation? If you are looking for an answer, I am afraid I do not have one. I do believe that when one is asked to write a letter on a mentee, you should state that you are wanting to know the results of the promotion and tenure committee. If there is not a promotion, this is a sign that the dyad should meet and plan how to improve the educator portfolio of the CE going forward. It is also important to know overall that your mentoring is making a difference, and only the mentee can tell you that, providing key feedback on what has gone well and what needs improving.

- Being asked to be a mentor is flattering and one should accept all requests. This is a tricky area as I have been approached by many residents, medical students and CEs to mentor them. Here is how I have resolved that dilemma: (1) I have never mentored more than 5 trainees and/or fellow CEs at a time, and even that number is very time-consuming. So, basically, if I have reached my limit on mentees, I do not accept more. (2) Sometimes there is not a good 'fit' between mentor and mentee and I point that out to the trainee or faculty, making general suggestions on how to proceed going forward. (3) Writing strong letters of recommendation are an integral part of being a mentor and if you peruse the trainee's/CE's CV and are unable to write a strong recommendation, you have to be honest regarding that issue. That doesn't mean that another mentor could not write a good letter for that person. It is important to interview any trainees and CEs asking for mentorship and making certain there is a good fit between you. For the most part, I have always accepted fellow CEs as mentees, helping them succeed and be recognized by peers in whatever area they chose to excel, a major focus for me and usually for them. Mentoring fellow CEs always was a priority to me and I did this locally and nationally. Many CEs nationally have said to me post-retirement what a wonderful mentor and role model I have been to them and this has been flattering as some of my experiences have been collaborating on papers, workshops and even conversations over coffee (I am humbled!). We don't always know how we have impacted people until they tell us!!! And as pointed out previously, we don't offer hear back from those whom we mentor.

- Not setting up ground rules about the mentoring process. So, when engaging people to accept as mentees, the CE should seek what the person wants from the relationship and what kind of help you might provide. Perhaps I am wrong, but I perceive that many trainees want someone to write a strong letter of recommendation for them regarding residency training or job offers and perhaps nothing else. That is far short of what I see a mentor potentially doing. The mentoring process may focus on gender issues, ES, administrative organization skills, and balancing life and academic responsibilities. Having the trainee identify strengths and weaknesses and areas to be addressed based on this reflection is important. Teaching that trainee to reflect and determine their own strengths and weaknesses is a life-long skill. Timelines are also important in that trainees and CEs are busy BUT there needs to be periodic meetings to examine progress in certain areas and how the trainee is doing health-wise, their professional development and personally. I have found the mentor has to assume the responsibility for setting up these meetings as trainees get 'lost' in doing other things. Some questions that might arise are how often meetings should occur, what format, how to best communicate between meetings, and who will set the agenda (ideally, the mentee) among other issues. It is probably safe to state that conflicts will arise (e.g., personal and family issues, academic responsibilities) that sometime preclude meeting as regularly as was determined by both parties. That, however, should not be an ongoing occurrence and if it is, might be a reason to end the relationship. Another reason to mutually end the relationship is when the mentee feels like he has accomplished the goal(s) set out initially and no longer perceives needing further mentorship. Finally, Janet Serwint, M.D., emeritus Professor of Pediatrics from Johns Hopkins, has described mentoring as 'Helping the mentee to understand that the journey is as important, and maybe more so, than the destination'.
- Discounting generational gaps between the dyad. Characteristics ascribed to specific generations are absolutely and somewhat frighteningly real, and what worked for one generation might not at all be applicable to others. Of course, this means refraining from being judgmental when listening to the mentee's goals and needs. I found a nice balance between my professional and personal life, with major strategies being getting to work very early and checking items off my to-do list before most colleagues arrived; and delegating tasks traditionally done by physicians to others. I made certain I was surrounded by capable people with

a good work ethic and who valued my search for excellence in all that I did. This model enabled me to think creatively and never have a static moment in my career. However, this path might not at all fit that of a junior mentee of today and I was careful in my mentoring to not impose what worked for me on someone else. It is fine to describe what worked for me in my career, **if asked**; but every mentee is unique in her needs and what she seeks from the mentor. It's fun revisiting those successes and sharing those secrets.. Nothing happened to me serendipitously; things followed a plan, which overall was that I wanted to make a difference in my career.

- Not setting goals from the start. It is important, in concert with the mentor, for the mentee to set goals for the relationship and for her career, short-term and hopefully longer-term. That should include personal issues, as they balance professional responsibilities with their professional life. A concern is that some idealistic CEs come to a medical center without clear goals although they know what part of the mission they like; e.g., patient care. That being the case, having that person determine how he will demonstrate excellence in that area and document that for his educator portfolio should be an important area on which to focus with the mentor. Of course, although this probably does not need to be stated, any conversations between the dyad are always confidential as part of their trusting relationship.

- Not reflecting on the relationship. As time goes on, there may be a reason to part ways, hopefully amiably as people change as do needs. The mentee may not live up to expectations in scheduling regular discussions with the mentor or in attaining goals she set up for herself. Maybe there is a message here but this should be discussed to tease out potential root causes of the behavior. As a mentor, one needs to be supportive and not judgmental of the mentee. However, when there are objective problems that are factual (not perceptions) about the mentee not achieving goals, revisiting the relationship is appropriate and either partner can determine that this is not working. Of course, there are times when the mentor is not perceived as value-added by the mentee and this is a reason to discontinue the relationship. That being said, it is not detrimental for the mentee to fail in some aspects of his work IF learning evolves from that failure. What would be unacceptable is ongoing failure to meet expectations set by the dyad.

- Pushing a personal agenda that worked for you. Of course, the mentee and you need to discuss what you think you can offer in the relationship, with the ultimate goal being that the mentee assumes independence in decision-making around goals. If indeed exploratory discussions reveal there is not a fit between the mentor and mentee, then it's clear the relationship should not be continued. Approaching this with a blueprint, cookie-cutter personal agenda is not what the mentee needs from us. Just as in teaching, CEs need to be facilitators of the process, allowing the mentee to take the lead and be proactive. It's all about the mentee's needs, not what worked for the mentor. When we see areas that concern us, we can state those but not be forceful in changing the mentee's mind once we have made our point. Encouraging the mentee to focus on whatever the goal(s) should be a major mantra of the mentor.

- All mentors represent their field. I remember a fourth medical student who determined that surgery would be her career goal. This was based on interacting with a surgeon during her surgical clerkship who was an amazing role model professionally and personally. She came to realize that all surgeons were not like the icon who influenced her and that he was not representative of his field in how he behaved. Making a career choice as a medical student or resident may mean sampling from many faculty, some of whom are mentors and others through brief clinical encounters. Mentors and mentees need to address this issue of how one would analyze the characteristics of a given field, enumerating what a day is like in the life of that faculty member and the kinds of candidates the field attracts.
- Mentoring is all work and adds another layer of responsibility for the mentor. No one ever said mentoring is easy, especially if the needs of one's mentees are significant. I've already stated that limiting the number of mentees is reasonable if one is at the entry to mid-levels of a CE. However, I must say that mentoring can be one of the most rewarding parts of being a CE. Seeing mentees succeed with your oversight can be so humbling to know you played some part in that success story. Obviously, the mentor's role may be the 'enzyme' that catalyzes the reaction; i.e., leading to that mentee's success. There are so many examples of this and many in my career revolved around trainees involved with my ES, leading to presentations at national meetings and then publication. For a lot of this work, we model how we do things in our professional and personal lives without necessarily vocalizing in describing those activities. The highest compliment can be that the mentee wants to emulate and be as successful as you are.
- Not being able to say 'no' when a potential mentee has an agenda that is not within your expertise. Having an initial fact-finding session with the potential mentee to determine if his/her needs are in-synch with the mentor's is very important going forward. The CE, upon hearing the mentee's story and needs, can make a decision on whether or not this dyad relationship will work effectively. I remember a senior medical student who requested I be her mentor and I was very hesitant. The major drawback for me was that I was aware that this woman had chosen surgery as her career choice and then backtracked and decided on pediatrics. In our initial 'intake', she related her personal family story regarding her sister, who was a quadriplegic from a car accident. At 13 years of age and part of a single parent family, she independently made the decision to leave school and commit to caring for her sister, eventually earning a G.E.D. degree and going on to college and medical school. I was so moved by her story of resilience that I accepted her as a mentee. Hearing her story, I felt a connection with her as she related how she got to where she was in life. Bottom line is to make certain you have the knowledge and skills to provide counseling to whatever mentees you accept in your practice and know some of their life experiences.
- Not sharing our 'failures' with mentees. As creative CEs exploring unknown areas, we predictably experience failures in our careers, causing us to reflect, recalibrate and reassess. Taking chances when working in unknown territory can result in failures, although that might not be the right description when initiatives are unsuccessful. These adventures can become learning opportunities going forward,

resulting in edited and successful projects. It should be apparent that we as mentors do not have all the answers and that should be divulged early on in the relationship with a mentee. Discussing these 'failed opportunities' as general teaching points with mentees humanizes us and presents a forum to verbalize these faux pas as a way to share our experiences. Whenever I had a project that did not produce what I expected, it was easy for me to say to myself that it was time to regroup, recalibrate and/or move on.

- Not establishing a formal ending to the relationship. The mentoring is almost never forever, at least in a formal context. Both parties can decide when the mentorship is no longer needed based on academic growth, confidence, life experiences, and when the mentor reflects that she no longer has knowledge and skills to enhance the career of the mentee. This point will happen at different times for many and represents a joint decision (in most cases) when to **formally** end the relationship. It would be unusual for both parties not to keep in touch even when this closure occurs, based on long, often intimate and rich interactions. The timing of this closure actually should be a talking point when the two agree to this relationship, making the decision more comfortable for both the mentee and mentor.
- Not taking care of oneself emotionally and/or physically. Ok, this comment does not fit into any of the above categories but probably is one of the most important if not the most important misadventure I have mentioned. I hope we have learned from the Covid pandemic what effect isolation, not feeling connected, decreased socialization, the overload of patients and depression have had on us going forward. Tending to our physical, nutritional and emotional health consciously is a habit to which we need to adhere. Carving out time to do something aerobic three times or so a week is a goal we should strive for. In addition, if we, our significant other or friends see our mental health somehow failing, we should know there are services available to put us on the right path to wellness. We cannot be there for our patients, colleagues and trainees if we ourselves are not well.

In summary this book focuses on misadventures in medical education and patient care, highlighting areas that can go wrong and how we as CEs can recognize those and turn those mistakes into successes. I hope the examples I use become niduses for further discussion with trainees and peers, perhaps generating additional topics I omitted for further rich discussions in numerous venues. Reflecting on our performance in education and patient care represents a willingness to examine what we can improve. I wrote this book with that end in mind. I wish you luck in your endeavors and remember that to err is human. Recognizing those errors and growing from that recognition is what makes faculty successful in their careers. Carpe diem, as Robin Williams said in Dead Poets.

# Reference

Choi, A. M.. K., Moon, J. E., Steinecke, A., Prescott, J. E. (2019). Developing a culture of mentorship to strengthen academic medical centers. *Academic Medicine, 94*(5), 630–633. https://doi.org/10.1097/ACM.0000000000002498